This is a great book for anyone interested in knowing the basics of how everything "down there" works, and that there are medical answers to most urological problems. As author Madeline Zech says, "If you own a vagina or a penis, you need to read this book!" In this amusing urology handbook, Zech argues that it's well past time for society to get over its discomfort regarding our plumbing system. She not only provides critical information about that system for both men and women but she also encourages readers to be proactive participants in keeping it healthy. A very educational and entertaining read!

– Kirkus Reviews

UROLOGY

The Ins and Outs Ups and Downs

Madeline Zech

This book is a must read for anyone who has "one" and all the functions that go with each "one". My daughter has done a great job putting urological problems and solutions into laymen terms for everyone to understand. This book is well written and entertaining, while still delivering solid information that is sure to help.

Paul Zech,
Her Dad

Every man and every woman in the world should know more about urologic conditions. It is through books like this that knowledge will be turned into better health.

Ian M. Thompson, Jr. M.D.
Member of Texas Urology Group
Former Chairman, Department of Urology, University of Texas San Antonio
Former President, American Urological Association Former President, American Board of Urology

This is a book about those urologic curiosities that both men AND women experience So be ready ladies - Madeline sheds a light in a simple manner on those urologic parts of your own with the hope that they can be helped should they go awry.

Mandie Tibball Svatek, M.D.
Associate Professor of Pediatrics, UT Health San Antonio, TX

UROLOGY

THE INS AND OUTS UPS AND DOWNS

MADELINE ZECH

ISBN 978-1-952114-75-5
eBook available wherever digital books are sold.

Cover Design: Aleksandar Petrovic, vajsman@gmail.com
Graphic Design: Goran Skakic, gskakic@gmail.com

Library of Congress Control Number: 2020902782
Printed in the United States of America

FOREWORD

The numbers are staggering, and nobody wants to talk about it. More than half the men in this country are affected at some point in their lives by erectile dysfunction. Too many men will be diagnosed with prostate cancer or have difficulty trying to pee.

Women are not far behind with persistent problems being sexually aroused, achieving orgasm or dealing with pain during sex. Mix it all together and you end up with a lack of desire.

Throw in plumbing problems like incontinence for both sexes and now you see the need to almost laugh and cry at the same time. But, don't do that or you might leak!

Although this is no laughing matter, urology will be the most entertaining conversation you will have with your closest friends. Throw in this book and you will laugh out loud, while at the same time getting the answers to how things down there get fixed. Find the answers to get your plumbing working again and regain your quality of life.

Regardless of your sexual orientation this book focuses on the function of penises and vaginas and how they can affect your quality of life.

In the end, we are all connected on the inside by our plumbing and all that goes with it. This reality with our human plumbing should give us all a healthy perspective on humanity. Urology is a basic reminder to work harder at being kind to everyone, no matter how different we think we may be. Urological struggles are an equalizer for the human race.

The author has been with a reconstructive urologist, "The Doctor". He has one of the busiest medical practices in town that has helped her to easily create a "Top 10 Type" list of the most prevalent urological problems for both men and women.

The author translates medical urological situations in a sensitive and humorous way.

This book is gentle enough for every man to read, funny enough for every woman to enjoy, and educational enough to give a copy to everyone you know. The author makes it safe and accepting to talk about all things urological and encourages you to embrace your plumbing.

CONTENTS

Final thoughts

Chapter 1

HOW DID THIS HAPPEN TO ME?

Let the journey begin to open your heart and mind

Here's my typical day:

- Erectile dysfunction inquiry on aisle 6 next to the whole wheat bread.
- Leaky vagina after orgasm question in the parking lot of the high school.
- Obvious prostate interruptions in the middle seat, Row 8, followed by an hour-long conversation about all the urinary trouble he's been having for the last two years.

And I love it all! Who knew that I could warm up to all things penis and vagina without blushing or breaking a sweat at the mere mention of those words? It is fascinating to me that perfect strangers somehow discover that I am married to the Doctor and ask for my help with their most intimate problems. I am not sure why people from all walks of life, and sometimes perfect strangers, would be brave enough to disclose their most personal urological issues to me. Perhaps it is because I am quick to share a smile or a quick friendly conversation? As a genuinely kind person who is always willing to help, I have had the most wonderful human experiences with people everywhere. Making human connections and showing love for other human beings is truly the best part of my life.

Throughout my days in my small town I am often spotted by the doctor's patients, both past and present. Just to give you an example of how it goes down, let me share with you what happens when I am innocently waiting for my coffee in line at Starbucks. While standing in line like everyone else, yearning for that first hot beverage of the day, I am bored and looking around and fidgeting on my smartphone. As I glance out the window, I see a familiar truck pull into the parking lot. As the gentleman gets out of his car, I know exactly who he is and remember when he shared with me his difficult urological situation in the same line at Starbucks. Immediately, I start praying that he will not head right for me and stop to ask another penis question that he wants me to run by the doctor.

I turn around quickly so he cannot see my face, and as I do, I run right smack into the bakery lady from our local grocery store, who was immediately happy to see me. My panic was only obvious to me as I managed to plaster on a warm and friendly smile to make her comfortable as she approached. She always makes it a point to seek me out at the grocery store to say hello, hug me as though I am her favorite daughter, and tell me how appreciative she is of the help. She recently told me she was scheduled to see the doctor and have her pelvic prolapse issue fixed. Today, it just happened to be in line at Starbucks.

Still in line for coffee, the bakery lady tells me that she had been to all of her appointments and was hopeful that the doctor was going to be able to fix the pelvic prolapse issue plaguing her for years.

I must admit that I do love people. It was the penis and vagina part of these encounters that always had me sweating and forced me to deal with my modesty. I have come to understand that this is simply another one of my shortcomings. I am not the doctor, but a woman taking care of kids and parents and a demanding household. This is no light load to carry in this lifetime. It can be tough when everyone in line at Starbucks is listening in, so the next time they see me, they too can come up and share their urological issues in hopes of finding help for either themselves or someone they love.

As the years have gone on and hundreds of people have approached me, it makes me stop and think how much pee is flowing on the planet. The volume of people that seek me out like a heat-seeking missile to access the man who can fix their pee problems has made me want to stand up and shout out to the world that there is help for your plumbing problems.

If anyone would have told me 20 years ago that this would be my life as the doctor's wife, I would have run the other direction and never looked back. I am now up to my neck in small-town living, where privacy is hard to come by and everyone somehow knows my connection to a reconstructive urologist who fixes penises and vaginas. I have been sucked into the vortex of all things urological. What has surprised me the most is that I know nothing about urology but have heard some great stories that have touched me in some way or flat out made me laugh.

Through all the human interactions and urological stories, I always remember how important it is to be kind and compassionate. As a result, I have learned a lot about urology along the way. However, I still secretly laugh Secretly laugh and ask the doctor and ask the Doctor what I think must be stupid questions about all things urology. He assures me that no question is stupid when it comes to trying to understand my own plumbing or his.

All this new knowledge in my head has led me to believe that perhaps I am just like everyone who approaches me with caution because this subject matter is not something that is normally discussed. I can relate to them and their potential stress about a urological medical condition.

Through this twisted path of kindness and urine, I have come to learn that I truly care, and I do love being able to help people from all walks of life in some small way, whether it has to do with pee pee or not.

So why do I open myself up to strangers and welcome their inquiries with a warm and friendly demeanor? Because I have come to learn something special about myself. I am a deep and loving soul, and I am learning that it is okay to talk about this, too.

This journey of finding myself through my random acts of kindness toward others is really a story about my love of helping and healing and making the world a better place one person at a time. I do care about people and I want people to know that they matter. I do that every time someone comes up to me for help with their urological problems. I take time out wherever I am and whatever I am doing to stop and listen.

It's not always convenient because most of the time I am trying to take care of my family. However, I understand that it takes tremendous courage to come up to me with such intimate information in an effort to somehow get help.

Perhaps open conversations about urology are one area where I can help to make a difference and help heal intimate relationships. When any close relationship is strained, it can result in stress and isolation. Urological problems can be incredibly isolating because it's not easy to talk about your pee or your penis or your vagina. Those three words alone can be devastating.

Without going to medical school, I have been put in a position where I believe I can have a positive impact on people's lives by simply being a directional sign with a friendly smile and a warm heart. I have learned a great deal through other people's urological problems as I try to connect them to the true healer, the Doctor. I am grateful for the opportunity to be kind in a way that will somehow make the world a better place one person, and one penis or one vagina, at a time.

So enough about me, let's get on with some urological stories and the fixes available for both men and women that can change lives for the better. We'll have some good laughs together while learning the truth about our own plumbing, what happens when it fails, and what to do about it.

Chapter 2

UROLOGICAL FOREPLAY

To share is to trust

The subject of urological problems is about as embarrassing to me as it gets. I am sure the same must be true for most of us who are not in the medical field. Let me preface this entire book with the fact that I am not a doctor nor do I claim to have any medical knowledge about the subjects that I am so bravely about to put into layman's terms so we can all better understand what these doctors already know.

You may wonder why I am writing this tell-all book. It is because for the last 20 years or so, I have been asked by hundreds of people to be the urological liaison between them, the ordinary citizen, and the doctor. At first it was like the blind leading the blind and we were both looking for the doctor and his knowledge. Hundreds of future patients, their spouses, or complete strangers have approached me as they tried to gain access to an appointment with the doctor or to find answers to an array of urological issues. It's funny when they speak to me as though I am the doctor. I have had more people tell me things I never wished to hear and there is no way to ever erase it from my mind. I had no earthly idea that the human body had so many issues. But I am not a doctor. I am simply an outsider, who happens to have a ringside seat next to the Doctor. This unusual setup has put me in a unique position on many occasions out in public and in every venue you can imagine.

Life with the Doctor has been a wild ride as I have become the conduit or the "secret door" to his services. It's as though I have been inducted into a secret society of magic treatments while attaining near-celebrity status in our small town because of the medical gifts the doctor bestows upon our community. My role in this partnership was not by choice or inclination. This new adventure into the world of urology and how it affects every single person at some point in their lifetime has humbled me and inspired me to help.

But in the beginning, I really had no clue what my the doctor really did as a physician because I had never seen a urologist myself. Some things you don't learn until you need to know. Especially subjects that are quite personal or embarrassing like urology.

Soon after we moved to town, local community members began to identify us as the family of the new urologist. It so happened that the doctor was the only guy in about a 400-mile radius who could provide certain specialized urological services. Our circle of acquaintances began to grow quickly, followed by inquiries about every urological problem imaginable. This was when my real education began.

For the first ten years of our marriage, I was absolutely perplexed as to how people knew who I was. They were complete strangers to me, and I had never spoken to them or met them formally. Evidently, people talk and look and quietly point fingers. I guess this is the only time it's a good thing. For me, it was a totally different experience as people were incredibly friendly and gracious when they approached me.

Here is a perfect example of what has happened countless times. While getting my oil changed at the car dealership, I thought I would go inside to the sales room and say hello to my car salesman. Let's call him John, for the sake of protecting his privacy. John informed me that he had been a patient of the doctor in the past and he had finally pieced together the fact that I was married to his doctor.

John was a proud Latino in his 60s whose professionalism and courtesy were always appreciated. He was extra happy to see me on this day, and I was happy to see him as always. He seemed to be in a talkative mood and went out of his way to offer me coffee, water and even donuts. Despite telling John that my car was finished getting a quick oil change and that it was ready and waiting for me, he just kept making pleasant conversation. Now remember, John is an older Latino, and in general, they are incredibly private when it comes to personal issues such as urology. It probably didn't make it any easier that I am a nice-looking lady, the last person he would want to confide in about an embarrassing pee problem.

After saying again that it was time for me to leave, John gently touched my elbow and said, "I have a question for you if you don't mind." I, of course, said, "sure thing, how can I help?" John started to tell me some of his symptoms, and as he started talking, small beads of sweat started to form on his forehead. John shared he had been peeing blood for about a month and had done the right thing by calling the doctor office for an appointment. But, he explained, he couldn't get in for the next three months. Sadly, this is a medically underserved community so there aren't enough doctors to help the total population here. I asked John if he wouldn't mind if I called the doctor on the spot and let him speak to him directly so they could discuss the issue and find out if this was an urgent matter.

I dialed up the Doctor and handed the phone over to John so he could explain his symptoms. Out of respect and privacy, I walked away pretending to be interested in all the new cars in the showroom. When the phone call was finished, John told me he was going to see the doctor the very next morning. You could visibly see his relief, and it felt great to be able to provide some support.

This same routine happens EVERYWHERE I GO. It can be at the post office, the grocery store, the tutoring studio, the gym, the golf course, the airport, the local park... it happens EVERYWHERE. I have decided to call this entire pre-appointment experience with strangers "Urological Foreplay." I don't know what else to call it. I get the dramatic buildup about all the urology problems, from every acquaintance or stranger in town, but I never get to hear the ending because I am not the doctor, and of course, the doctor never talks about his patients. He just tells me if I want to know, I will have to ask the patient. I would never go back and ask a patient if they were still peeing blood. Holy heck, I am sweating as much as they are when listening to their urological problems, and I am not even the one with the problem! Who knew that urology foreplay could make both parties sweat?

As the wife of the Doctor, I learned immediately how to keep a straight face and act as though every word these people were saying was the most important thing I had ever heard. I always reacted calmly, but I was completely out of my league about what to say. So I would simply say, "Let me call the doctor so he can help you." Upon escaping these situations, I would frantically search for somewhere private to regroup and collect my thoughts, wondering why people were so willing to tell me unbelievably personal things.

Playing this role as the Doctor's wife did not come without mistakes on my part, many of them over the years, as the doctor has repeatedly emphasized how sensitive urological issues are for all patients.

For some reason, the prostate is always at the top of the list. I often wondered why this subject got such respect and would especially wonder why every year when my annual exam came around it seemed to be public information. The entire staff in the office always knew I was married to the Doctor and the gynecologist would even interrogate me during the examination about what urological miracles the doctor was currently performing. The visit would always end with, "I should really give the doctor a call because it's time for my prostate exam." I really did not need to know this! Yet another example of why opening the discussion about urology does matter.

Another thing I have learned is that almost all your urological problems can be solved. But the Doctor tells me that the average patient will wait years after symptoms start before coming to see him because they are often embarrassed or do not realize there is help available for them. So they just suffer through it and have simply learned to live with their problem. Shocking, sad, and so unnecessary.

My own mother was a perfect example of this denial and refusal to ask for help. Struggling with urinary incontinence for 30 years after having eight children, she planned her daily life around a map of toilets in town for immediate access as needed. The doctor finally said enough is enough and insisted on bringing her in for a treatment plan. She was amazed to learn that a simple surgery would change everything and now wishes she had done it decades ago. Mom was beyond thrilled with her newfound freedom.

With all of this exposure to people agonizing over urinary problems, I decided it is time to share what I have learned from the Doctor so we can all talk about it in a way that will reduce the humiliation and embarrassment. When I started telling people close to me about writing this book, the positive responses and eagerness for the information were overwhelming. The most common problems among men, women, and youth are more than enough for this book and an entire series going forward.

The secrets of the Doctor are really the things that everyone not only wants to know but needs to know. As the doctor always says, "Every single person at some point in their life will need a urologist." Those are very intimidating words until you come to learn the value of what a urologist can do to restore your quality of life. I have seen it with my own eyes.

Now a confession: I will tell you right now that the doctor is not at all happy, I am writing this book and putting it out into the world. First, because it is not academic or highly technical, like a medical textbook, with all those details none of us understand. Urology is a serious business to him, and he does not consider any of these related subjects funny. Nor is he thrilled with the fact that his wife is about to share secrets from the crypt about our sexual health as individuals and as a couple. It has become clear to me this entire subject is not only taboo for the public, but also uncomfortable for the Doctor. All the more reason to start the conversation so the door may be opened to all things urology and knowing how to get help when your personal plumbing malfunctions.

It has been an honor to serve in my capacity as the wife of the Doctor and I hope the information provided on the pages to come continues that contribution. So, sit back and join me in learning about a subject both terrifying and humanizing all at the same time, while maintaining your sense of humor.

Chapter 3

FROM THE MILITARY TO SMALL TOWN USA

The unknown is yet to be discovered

I met the doctor while living in Seattle when he was stationed at Ft. Lewis, Washington. It was truly love at first sight for me. I had no idea who this guy really was, but I knew I was going to marry him from the first date. Little did I know all that would follow.

Happily working as a woman in the world of computers while he was in the Army serving our great nation, somehow our lives came together. We eloped to Honolulu, where we were married in the Fort DeRussy chapel by a Special Forces soldier who was also a chaplain.

Still living in Seattle, our first child was born nine months after that – a beautiful boy. Just ten days later, we moved cross-country to small town USA and started a new adventure together, leaving both the military and the corporate craziness behind. The doctor was focused on practicing medicine in a bicultural, medically underserved community with sunshine, while I was determined to be a stay-at-home mom and care for our new family.

Soon, baby number two arrived for us – a beautiful little girl. We were now a family of four and having children thrust us into the world of playgroups and preschools where all the mommies would gather. This new introduction to the world of moms and babies was far more than just that though. It would be the emergence of my role as the Doctor's wife. No surprise, nearly all of them had husbands, and every single one of them had gone through childbirth. These life experiences are often the onset of multiple urological issues for both men and women. Women can have difficulties during delivery that can be the start of urological concerns. Men tend to gain weight when wives are pregnant and that in turn leads to the possibility of high blood pressure or diabetes. Weight gain, high blood pressure, and diabetes in men take us directly to potential problems with the penis.

Chapter 4

PENIS PASSION AND VAGINA NAVIGATION

Passion has no rules

Why on earth would anyone want to spend their life fixing penises and vaginas? This is a valid question for someone like me, who simply enjoys computers, but you wouldn't believe how often this subject comes up. It's no small question when you stop and consider that the Doctor is so specialized in this field that he spent 15 years of his life studying penises and vaginas along with other urological anatomy. Four years of pre-med in college, four years of medical school, six years in residency, and one year in fellowship training. That is 15 years of training on how to fix a penis or vagina and all the plumbing that goes with each one. Now just stop and think about that for a minute. It's almost impossible to understand that kind of dedication until you become a patient of the Doctor and experience the magic of having your urological problem solved.

This brings to mind a memory of when my son was in kindergarten. We have always spoken to our children in medical terms for obvious reasons. It is technically correct, as it is merely anatomy. When the children were younger, they always wanted to know where papa was and why he was not home. I had to explain to them that he was fixing people. They would ask what papa was fixing and I would always tell them that he was fixing broken penises and vaginas so people could go pee pee like us. No big deal, right? Well, guess again.

When the kindergarten teacher asked each of her students what their parents did for a living, you can imagine the answer that came out of my son's mouth: a technically correct answer. The principal then called to report that my son had a potty mouth! I proceeded to educate the principal that he, too, had a penis that would one day need to be fixed by a Doctor of urology so either stop asking the kids about their parents' profession or be prepared for the answer. By the way, the principal was a priest at the Catholic school.

So why become a Doctor? The answer is almost boring; his father was also a Doctor. Yep, it's that simple. He wanted to be just like his father! The Doctor's father would be considered a general urologist; however, the Doctor took it a step further and became sub-specialized in the same field and focused on Female Pelvic Medicine and Reconstructive Surgery, which is just one of the sub-specialties within urology.

Evidently, there are different types of urologists that sub-specialize which is a very important fact to know, especially if you need a specialized Doctor like a urologist. The Doctor can also do general urology, but being so specialized, it makes more sense to use his time and skills to take on the more complicated reconstructive cases in which he was trained to handle.

General urologists are usually the place to start for any problems you may be having down there. They evaluate, diagnose, and treat all the most common urological issues such as vasectomies, circumcisions, infections, and prostate conditions. General urologists will refer you to a sub-specialist when indicated for specific situations outside their expertise.

A reconstructive urologist like the Doctor is the guy who rebuilds everything down there in case you suffer any trauma to the pelvic area or have physical abnormalities that interfere with good pee flow. The other types of urologists are pediatric urologists, which handle anyone under 18, and uro-oncologists, which handle all urological cancers. There is also the endo-urologist, which handles minimally invasive surgery and specializes in types of stone disease. They are also good with endoscopic surgery and robotic surgery, which are both minimally invasive. There are also urologists that specialize in sexual medicine and infertility. This specialty is a separate fellowship training and almost a new frontier of information in the world of urology. There is the more dramatic sub-specialty of urological trauma and reconstruction. This surgeon fixes you if you get shot, run over, or even hit by a bus. They are the cleanup crew. A urological trauma surgeon or a reconstructive urologist are the only type of urologist that can put your plumbing back together and in good working order.

Every patient should become thoroughly educated about their diagnosis, treatment options, and the best type of urologist for that particular problem. This allows you to participate fully with the doctor in determining the best course of treatment. Researching qualifications of the doctor, how often he has treated your type of condition, and any specific training he has received with the type of surgery you may need will go a long way toward making you more comfortable about a good outcome.

If this explanation of the various doctors working in urology has left you totally confused about the best way to go, let's look at an analogy using a baseball team with all of its specialty players. Each position on the team is specifically trained to do a highly skilled and specific job, but all within the game of baseball. The same concept is true in the world of urology; each specialist has a particular role to play on the team working to improve your plumbing.

In baseball, the pitcher pitches, the catcher calls the pitches and catches, and the first baseman is like the laser-focused player with the giant baseball glove who somehow seems to snag every single ball whizzing in at

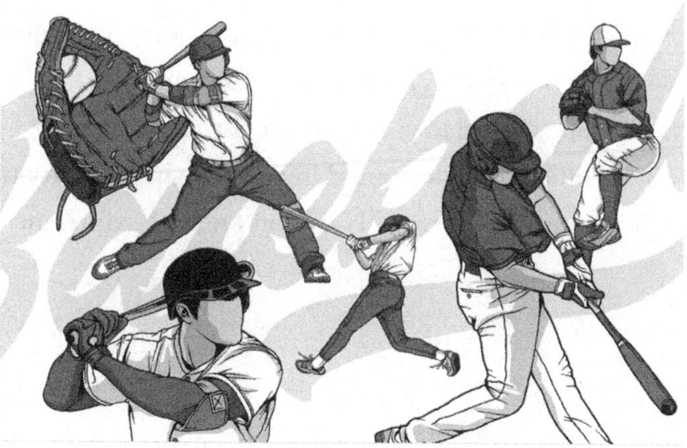

9,000 mph. But, just imagine the equipment manager out there covering first base instead; his expertise in bats, gloves, and balls is nearly worthless in stopping a line drive headed his way. The same is true with general urologists; some are like general managers overseeing the big picture and choosing the most qualified players for each situation in the game. These general urologists play the same roles by providing a wide range of fundamental services for patients but always call in highly specialized players for the skilled positions that require more complex treatments.

Bottom line: it matters who takes care of you! So, be bold in getting the information you need to be sure you are in the best possible hands for your condition. Don't let the equipment manager try to tell you he is now a pitcher. That is your job to investigate the qualifications of your urologist. Know their training and what position they are highly skilled at and capable of performing. This same investigation needs to be applied to your gynecologist, as they are usually not qualified to handle anything urology but may try to convince you differently. Now you know the difference.

Chapter 5

PENIS PRESSURES IN SOCIETY

Acceptance starts from within

Whether you are the penis owner or the penis recipient, this is a hugely delicate subject. Pondering why a man's penis is the most important thing in the world to him is a brave endeavor for any woman to embark upon. It is hard for women to relate and an uncommon question for a woman to ask of any man. This is because a woman's vagina is NOT the most important thing to her.

However, if you bring up the subject of the penis to anyone, man or woman, you will definitely get some type of reaction. From penis jokes to penis injuries, just the thought will usually cause a man to unknowingly cross his legs or cup his testicles to protect his jewels.

Women will chuckle at most penis jokes and roll their eyes like they know all about the penis and the power it holds, especially if it is small or experiencing dysfunction. This is where the weaponizing of the penis has come into play, forcing men to "measure up" or face the ridicule and shame of penis failure. The reality is that it's not funny at all. However, because most people are embarrassed to talk about the penis, humor often seems like a safe place and a way to deal with their discomfort.

The penis pressure and expectations that society puts on men are totally unrealistic. Let's just start there. You have enough blood for your brain OR your penis, but never enough for both! However, you can't get a man to believe this because society doesn't allow it. He is expected to effortlessly have an erection and be an amazing lover. A "real" man is also expected to have a huge penis. Because of these unspoken expectations, this is how many men measure themselves and their value in society.

When a man cannot get an erection or do the act, it is a deeply traumatic experience. This trauma greatly affects a man's mind and confidence. It is magnified when a man has a lover that is no longer supportive during this traumatic experience and may even leave him over it. Sadly, this is the outcome of sexual dysfunction more often than not.

This is where the jokes start about men and their hot sports cars in an effort to compensate for the inability to perform or lack of penis size. These jokes often have a grain of truth in them but are also very hurtful to those who are suffering.

Chapter 6

MY IMPOTENT MARRIAGE

Love enough to let go

So why am I bringing up the scariest thing that can happen to a man? Well, it took being married to the Doctor to finally help me understand why my first husband became impotent.

I was previously married to an amazing guy who was 12 years older than me. We had been married for several years and it was a wonderful time in my life. He came from a family that had serious cardiac disease. The DNA in his family was missing the gene that manufactures HDL, known as the good cholesterol. All that meant was when they ate something fatty like bacon, they did not have any of the good cholesterol to rid the body of the bad cholesterol. The only way to manufacture HDL was to exercise excessively. Although we lived a healthy lifestyle, the inevitable finally caught up to him.

Gradually, and prior to his first heart attack, I had noticed subtle changes in his performance in the bedroom. I noticed that he had a very hard time getting and maintaining an erection. My initial fear was that it might be me, which was part of the insecurity for being a young wife. At the time, it was not widely known in the medical community that the ability to get or maintain an erection had anything to do with a potential cardiac event.

Several years went by with this condition, and luckily, we enjoyed each other's company very much and found ways to "ignore" the problem with different ways of maintaining intimacy in our marriage. Then one day it happened. He was 42 just like his father who also had a massive heart attack at that age. Luckily, he was able to make it to the hospital where they were able to treat him and save his life. However, this heart attack rendered him completely impotent.

The next two years or so were an emotionally difficult time for both of us. He felt as though he was no longer a man. The fact that I was so much younger probably made it even more difficult for him and I am sure he felt more pressure to perform. I tried to reassure him, that he was my best friend and my forever partner no matter what. I loved him deeply and would never leave just because he could not maintain an erection.

As time went on, he pushed himself away from me and away from everyone. He spent more time at work and was easily agitated, frustrated, and very unhappy. Finally, he asked me to leave. I pleaded with him to let more time pass and we would figure things out together. But he simply said I needed to go. I told him that if that was how he truly felt, I loved him enough to let him go. Telling me it was what he wanted and needed, I walked away after a dozen years together with just my clothes and some heirlooms from my grandmother.

I had never stopped loving my first husband and spent the next several years grieving the loss of a great love and lover. The entire experience of going through a failed marriage due to impotence gave me a deep understanding and compassion of the toll it takes on a man and his family. I learned from a woman's perspective on what it can do. Impotence robs a man of everything he believes is required to make him a man, even though as a woman, I know differently.

There was nothing I could do to convince my first husband to just let me love him. He wouldn't have it. As I reflect back on that now, I suspect that asking me to leave was his way of dealing with the anger and humiliation of not being able to perform in the bedroom. It is impossible to truly stand in someone else's shoes. However, it is possible to show love and compassion in a way that is best for that person, even if it means letting them go because they asked you to do so.

As I have moved through life and reflected on the impact of erectile dysfunction and how it has affected my life, I have learned from the Doctor that there are solutions and technologies available that can save relationships. Erectile dysfunction is highly damaging to both partners and requires the help of professionals to help guide you through the gauntlet of care required to save both your health and your marriage.

The connection between sexual function and cardiac health has now been well established since the time my first husband and I paid the price of impotence in a marriage. In hindsight, it makes me sad and a bit angry that no erectile dysfunction treatment options were offered during his ongoing recovery from the heart attack. His cardiologist should have sent us to a urologist for an evaluation and help. In my mind, cardiologists and urologists should work as teams in men's health clinics to specialize in the body where there's also a psychologist on staff to support the couple through such a difficult time.

Today, thanks to the TV commercials, everyone knows all about the pills available for men suffering from erectile dysfunction. But no one ever talks about the various penile prostheses that are a treatment option. Just the terminology alone sounds both exciting and intimidating. If you have personally struggled with erectile dysfunction issues, it's probably not something you would readily think about. Otherwise, you would definitely want to know about every option available to help you get your manhood back in working order. As an outsider to the medical world, I had no idea there were so many options for help with erectile dysfunction.

Chapter 7

WHERE THE HELL IS MY AWESOME WOOD?

Inquiring minds find answers

One of the biggest perceptions of erectile dysfunction is the loss of your "manhood." The association is "oh my god, I am lesser of a man, or I am no longer a man." The social pressure and shame associated with erectile dysfunction are further compounded for the man if there is a pre-existing unhealthy relationship with his partner. If the wife is not interested in working through this problem or verbalizes that he is no longer a "man," there is a good chance the relationship will end. She may also leave him and take their children. Or she may cheat on him because he's not able to perform. But, if the wife is understanding and sensitive in supporting the husband's pursuit of treatment, their partnership can often continue to thrive. In reality, it's just a temporary situation that can be solved.

Now, you may think that no one would be so cruel as to actually tell her partner he is "no longer a man," but the doctor tells me that in his practice it is actually about 75% of women who will react this way when erectile dysfunction enters the relationship. This is especially true if the wife is significantly younger.

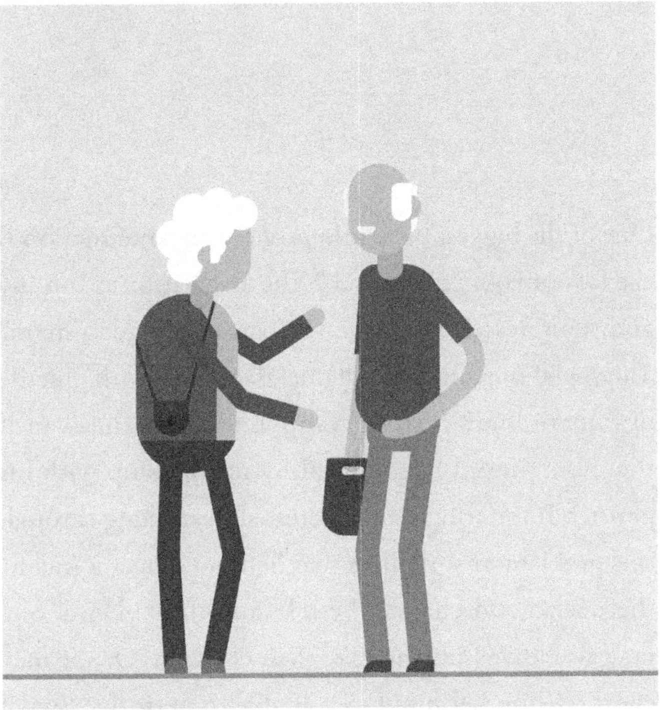

For those of you women who are reading this book and are remembering how poorly you treated a man experiencing this problem, you will see in the upcoming chapters that women can have their own sexual issues as they age including pelvic prolapse and incontinence during sex. Yes, you are probably going to pee all over yourself during an orgasm. So it is wise for all of us to reflect on being kind, supportive, and accepting of our partners as we all inevitably face health challenges. Tackling the problems as a team and seeking medical advice is the right path for getting a positive result.

This is where "The Doctor," steps in to make the world a more compassionate place for the male souls and the married couples who are brave enough and wise enough to come to his office for help. For the man whose wife left him for some younger guy with an erection, there is a pot of gold at the end of this rainbow. The Doctor has a beautiful answer for him. He assures the patient that not only is his erection problem going to be solved, but he will be even better than before and will find someone special to enjoy it with him. The terrified patient hears that he is not broken, just temporarily sidelined, and the previous partner did not deserve him.

Helpful hint: never refer to the problem as a "broken penis" because that whole concept is very disturbing to the man. I learned this when I asked the Doctor how a man could mentally get over having a broken penis. The Doctor immediately corrected me and told me to never ever say "broken penis." Ladies, pay attention to this very important message. It will save you a lot of unnecessary emotional and mental stress from your husband. The proper term to use when identifying a problem achieving erections is to simply identify it as a temporary situation and to seek treatment from a qualified urologist ASAP!

The success rate for fixing erectile dysfunction is very high. There are many treatment options to regain or improve erections relatively quickly. As it turns out, the number one most effective treatment is medication. There are currently five different medications that work for erectile dysfunction. Two of the drugs are available in a generic form that makes it more affordable and possible for most men to achieve an erection. You no longer need to pay $50.00 a pill.

The first option to treat erectile dysfunction include the following drugs: Viagra and Cialis (both in generic form), Stendra, and Levitra. You can now get 10 to 20 pills for under $100.00, whereas before it was approximately $50.00 per pill and most insurances did not cover it. Two of these drugs can also be compounded by your local pharmacist, reducing the cost even further.

There are other drugs that come in forms of injections or penile suppositories if the above medications don't work or your health conditions don't allow. Those other alternatives are alprostadil as a urethral suppository, which means it goes in the pee hole, or an injectable form called Trimix-gel, which is injected into the penis. This is a mixture of three medications, which include prostaglandin, papaverine, and phentolamine. This can only be injected directly into the penis. Although this sounds painful, the results can be very satisfactory. Another option is the vacuum erection device, which is exactly like it sounds. It sucks the blood right into the penis shaft and gives you a rock-hard erection. Once the erection is achieved, you simply slide the ring from the device onto the base of the penis shaft and you are ready to rock n roll.

These are the majority of solutions that are provided to patients initially. Most of them work very well, and at least one of these options will provide satisfactory results. If the above-mentioned solutions fail to work for you, or are not satisfactory, we have the ultimate solution in the next chapter that is covered by the majority of insurances, including Medicare. Just keep reading.

And a note to the woman who stood by her man through this traumatizing experience: I would bet $100.00 that you are more emotionally fulfilled, sexually satisfied, and more deeply in love with your partner because of overcoming erectile dysfunction together. You most likely have a new and deep appreciation for his erection. I would also lay another $100.00 bill on the table that your husband has a deep and profound love for you, as well as a desire to satisfy you in ways that neither of you could have ever imagined.

Chapter 8

PREMATURE EJACULATION THE ONE MINUTE WONDER!

Control has its Place and Time

This is a conversation that no man wants to discuss, and almost every woman has been the recipient of: Premature ejaculation! This topic has two different points of view: one from the woman, and one from the man. Men will almost never admit to the fact that they have experienced premature ejaculation, yet it is one of the top searched terms on the internet for sexual dysfunction topics. Women hear the term "premature ejaculation," and will almost always roll their eyes as they remember the time when they wanted it so badly, and their partner couldn't deliver. This is why relationships are challenged in ways that most people will never discuss, yet this can be a deal breaker in some cases.

Premature ejaculation may occur in many men, at some point in their lives. It tends to show up after long periods of abstinence or during very stressful times in life. Every man who is sexually active has experienced this difficult moment but will almost never admit to it as it is seen as a failure in the bedroom by men. This is only because it is that moment in a sexual encounter that is the most anticipated and sought-after delight. A man wants to satisfy his partner with this "explosion," and the woman is more than happy to receive it. Timing is everything and when your timing is off it can take the most magical moment and make it completely awkward without any warning.

It is important to remember that for many men, ejaculation is a part of orgasmic pleasure and a necessity for procreation. Furthermore, the inability to ejaculate at the "right time" can create a weakened sense of masculinity and interfere with the pleasure from an orgasm. It's important to remember that some men actually enjoy seeing their semen and can be agitated when the icing on the cake (ejaculate) is missing. For women and their ideas about ejaculate, I am sad to report that there is very little published data about females and their ideas about how sexual enjoyment is derived from their partner's climax ejaculation. I have several girlfriends, who definitely believe that ejaculation itself is an important part of their sexual desires and satisfaction.

You are only on the 3rd paragraph for this chapter, and I know that I have your full attention for this "taboo" subject. Think about that! More importantly, why aren't we talking about this? The great news is that this is another urological condition that is treatable!

Just so we are clear about how ejaculation occurs and why the stresses of life can get in the way, it's important to understand how your human plumbing works to achieve this Olympic moment. Ejaculation is controlled by the central nervous system. When men are aroused sexually, signals are sent to strategic parts of your body from the brain. When men get excited or see something they like sexually, messages are sent from your brain down to your zipper or what professionals would call the reproductive organs. This broadcast message is what gets the "General" to stand at attention and signal the troops to get ready to "fire," or ejaculate. Just to complicate the subject a little bit more, there are 2 types of premature ejaculation that are clinically defined.

Right now, you must be wondering how the simple subject of premature ejaculation can be defined, and how can we dig any deeper into a pretty obvious situation. Well, there can be several factors that create this "moment", and it takes a board-certified urologist to help you work through the possibilities so he or she can solve your issue.

The first type is called "Lifelong Premature Ejaculation" and the medical field defines this as poor ejaculatory control and ejaculation within about 2 minutes of initiation of penetrative sex that has been present since you became sexually active. Basically, when the tip of your penis receives stimulation of any kind and you are unable to control the ability to time your ejaculation. Goodbye Charlie!

The second type of premature ejaculation is called "Acquired Premature Ejaculation". This is defined as a consistently poor ejaculator control that happens much quicker than you experienced in previous sexual encounters during penetrative sex.

The good news is that regardless of either type of premature ejaculation condition, both are treated in a similar manner with a good measure of success. The only difficult part about treating premature ejaculation is saying this out loud to your doctor. This is the time when you know you are your own worst enemy because it is so difficult to talk about this subject. Perhaps this is why it is one of the most searched terms on the internet! It seems that most of the men in the world would rather seek the answer to their premature ejaculation problem in the privacy of their own computer.

Let me remind anyone reading this book that you can never SHOCK A UROLOGIST! They have spent their life learning how to solve your urological problem and have made it their mission to help you with yours! So with this thought in mind, pick up the phone and call your board-certified urologist and get started on the path to perfect timing.

So let's get to the good stuff! How do we treat premature ejaculation? You won't believe me, but it is almost as simple as changing positions, taking medication, applying a topical cream, or even talking to a sex therapist to gain a successful mental approach to your sexual thoughts. When you finally get the courage to seek treatment, your doctor is going to do a simple medical assessment, relationship assessment, and ask a few questions about your sexual history. Then they will perform a physical exam to evaluate if there are any clues about why you may be experiencing premature ejaculation. The solution can be a bit more involved for those that may need the help of a mental health professional with expertise in sexual health, but the end result will be the development of "perfect timing!"

As you start to practice your new skill, like with most things, you may need to adjust as you go along. Your doctor may suggest an adjustment to your medication depending on how you respond to either the oral or topical medications. You may also want to continue the conversation with your mental health professional in an effort to continue developing a healthy sexual thought process that allows you truly enjoy a satisfying sexual relationship.

If your doctor recommends a medication it is often a medication called Selective Serotonin Reuptake Inhibitor (SSRI), which is a low dose of an anti-depressant. This kind of medication is used to increase the level of serotonin, which is a neurotransmitter in the brain. This is the hormone that makes us feel good. The idea is to take this medication prescribed by your urologist, in an effort to slow down the ejaculatory event. The other option is a topical penile anesthetic such as lidocaine, which will slightly numb the penis tip and shaft in an effort to slow down ejaculation. You simply remove the lidocaine gel prior to insertion so that your partner does not lose their sensation. The end result is another well-timed event!

Now that you know you are not the only man on the planet who has experienced this urological issue, perhaps you will pick up the phone and call your board-certified urologist to come up with a game plan that works for you. This issue has many triggers and once you understand why this is happening to you, there are solutions for you to implement. Take this book with you to your doctor and start the discussion about how to solve premature ejaculation. Be prepared with a medication on hand for that special moment in case it was one of those days that was simply difficult and stressful. Premature ejaculation is a condition that comes and goes (pardon the pun), along with all the stresses and concerns that life throws at us.

Chapter 9

PENILE PROSTHESIS – YES, IT'S REAL AND IT WORKS!

The possibilities wake the soul

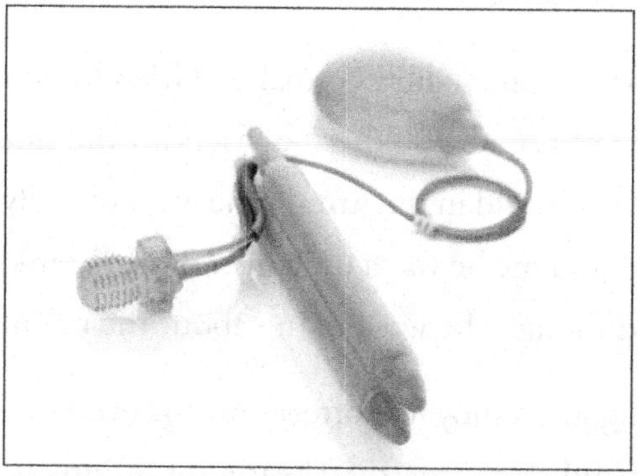

AMS Penile Prosthesis

Photos Courtesy of Boston Scientific

The Doctor is one of the top installers of the AMS inflatable penile prosthesis in Texas. Yes, this is an entire section about the inflatable penile prosthesis. They are real and they do work! This is the next step up for achieving an erection if the previous methods were not successful for you.

My first exposure to the phrase "inflatable penile prosthesis" happened when I took the Doctor home to meet my five brothers without him knowing that he was about to make the family introduction. I did not tell the Doctor about this family gathering because his nature is to over prepare for everything. I thought it would be better if this were an informal introduction with no preparation. Little did I know that my five brothers would have a million questions about everything "penis" related. These were my brothers after all, and somehow, I never realized they even owned a penis until my Doctor boyfriend showed up for dinner that day.

Initially, everyone was incredibly cordial and friendly and very welcoming of my new soldier boyfriend. I did not realize exactly what he did in the Army as he was not really a talker. He had told me he was a urologist. But I "heard" neurologist and thought he was talking about the brain.

It was a relaxing and enjoyable afternoon for everyone to be together, and of course, there was a lot of interest in the man I brought for dinner. Everyone assumed this must be the real deal, and soon my brother Dennis asked the first question of the Doctor. "So, Henry, how do you like being in the Army? That answer was obvious as he was very proud of his service to our country. And then the next question was asked. "So, what do you do in the Army?" The Doctor said, "I am a urologist." The standard response for most people is that they are sure they heard "neurologist", or they are either unfamiliar or terrified or embarrassed to acknowledge they heard "urologist."

Dennis then tried to get clarification on the new boyfriend's profession, so he asked him what kind of things a urologist does. This was a loaded question at a table with five of my brothers.

The Doctor was more than happy to share some of the things that he loves to do, which included dealing with incontinence, prostate issues, pelvic prolapse, and of course the crescendo, inflatable penile prosthesis!

This got everyone's attention as Dennis continued with the questions. "Penile prosthesis? How do those work anyway?"

Now this is the million-dollar question for several reasons because everybody wants to know about an inflatable penile prosthesis. It's the male insurance policy of a lifetime. It is the plan C in case plan A and B fail. Plan A is the "hot chick effect," plan B is "Viagra," and plan C is the secret device that everyone wants to hear about.

So, let's get started on the inflatable penile prosthesis from the wife's perspective. It all began one day in the garage as the Doctor was getting ready to leave for work and I was helping him take his things to his car. When he opened the trunk, I was shocked to see two cases of pills. One was Viagra and the other was Cialis. I also noticed other boxes which seemed very mysterious to me.

I first commented that having two cases of drugs in the trunk of his car would get him in big trouble if he were to get pulled over by the police for any reason. The Doctor said if he were to get pulled over and the cop were to see two cases of erectile dysfunction drugs, the Doctor would have an instant new best friend. I assured him that would not be the case if it were a female cop!

Then I just had to inquire about the other boxes which could be very intimidating or very exciting. One was labeled "AMS 700™ LGX Penile Prosthesis" which sounded like something out of a James Bond movie. There were two other boxes next to the first and were labeled "AMS 700™ CX Penile Prosthesis" and "AMS 700™ CXR Penile Prosthesis." My first thought was "Holy crap, you can pick your preferred model!"

I reached for the enticing box as if it were the jewel of the Nile and asked the doctor, "What the hell is this?" The doctor quickly reached out and gingerly took it from my hands. "Be careful with that! That is an inflatable penile prosthesis worth about $10,000." Now being the wife with all the questions and a pure talent for being direct, I asked why it was so big and how the heck did it fit inside a man's penis? The Doctor proceeds to pull out his index finger as though it were a penis and begins to explain how the device fits inside the penis shaft and connects to a tiny pump inside the testicle that will magically inflate the penis to a glorious angle of approximately 180 degrees when installed properly.

So what was up with the other two boxes with different model numbers? The Doctor informed me the three models of inflatable penile prostheses each have very specific purposes.

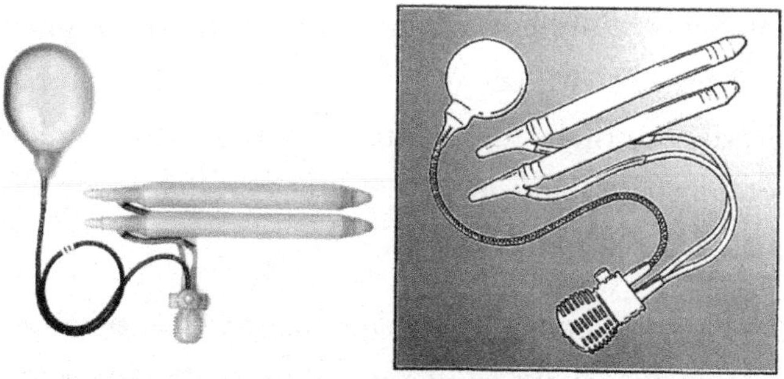

Photos Courtesy of Boston Scientific

Now because I am not a doctor and simply the hot sexy wife of the doctor, this is what I think I heard him say about the items in his trunk...

The first magic box, AMS 700 LGX Penile Prosthesis, is the most commonly used model. This is a 3-piece inflatable unit that is most commonly used for patients with a penis size of 20 cm or less. Now one question that everybody always asks, including me, is what size is the average penis? Is there an answer to this age-old question? Well, in the world of urology, where devices are used for medical conditions like erectile dysfunction, there is an answer! The average size of a penis in the doctor's opinion and experience is approximately 18 cm. Now before you pull out your smart phone and try to convert this magic number, let me help you out. This would be an erection of approximately 7.08661 inches. Everyone reading this book right now is probably happy and relieved to learn the average size of the doctor's patient base. This can probably be applied across all urology practices around the globe. Heck, you can almost confirm it because the penile prosthesis manufacturers have invested millions of dollars in these devices and they need to know what sizes will sell!

In the past, a prosthesis would just give you rigidity, or simply put, "make you hard." With the AMS 700 LGX Penile Prosthesis, it is designed to not only give you rigidity, but to also expand and give you 1 to 2 more centimeters in length, while also giving you more girth the more you use it. The reservoir in this 3-piece component allows the surgeon to add saline solution, which is simply done during installation. The amount of saline solution added is decided upon by your urologist to help you achieve an erection that is right for you. I asked the Doctor if you could add extra saline solution to the reservoir to get a bigger penis and the answer was no.

The AMS 700™ CX Penile Prosthesis is a more appropriate choice for the bigger penis because it gives a more rigid erection. The amount of fluid placed in the reservoir is slightly more and allows for more volume to be added and pumped into the cylinder and inflates in girth helping to achieve your new erection. Any patient that is greater than 20 cm would opt for this model. Just so everyone knows, this model is less commonly used.

The AMS 700™ CXR Penile Prosthesis is for the smaller penis. No judgment, just a solution that works wonders and also inflates in girth to give you maximum results.

After the discovery in the trunk of the doctor's car, I became even more curious about why there were such a variety of devices and how they actually looked. It just seemed to me that a man's penis was incredibly fragile and anything that appeared as large as what I thought I saw in the trunk of the doctor's car just did not add up. I decided to do a bit more investigating on my own, and over time, made many inquiries to the Doctor. He wondered why I had so much interest in the penile prosthesis and I assured him that I was not looking to make any recommendations for his penis and that all was well at the moment. What I learned is that there is an entire lineup of devices that help with most physical impairments that may get in the way of achieving an erection and/or managing an erection.

Because my the doctor prefers to work with the penile prosthesis from Boston Scientific, I felt most comfortable approaching the company and asking them for more information. The following is a lineup of penile implants made by Boston Scientific and it turns out they do indeed offer a variety of solutions for every man. As you will see, these devices are simple in nature and create a variety of solutions. The goal was to offer devices that can be operated by men who have manual dexterity (the inflatable variety) and devices for men who do not have manual dexterity (semi rigid). The following information and graphics are courtesy of Boston Scientific, who have been very supportive of my project to write this book in an effort to help people understand how a urologist can improve your quality of life.

The Boston Scientific AMS Penile Prosthesis Product Line includes the following implantable prosthetic devices:

AMS 700™ CX with MS Pump™ Penile Prosthesis – for the bigger penis

AMS 700™ CXR with MS Pump™ Penile Prosthesis – for the smaller penis

AMS 700 LGX with MS Pump™ Penile Prosthesis – the most commonly used model

The reservoir stores the fluid that fills and expands the penile cylinders. The patient operates the pump to inflate or deflate the system. The cylinders are inflated by multiple squeezes of the pump, which transfers fluid from the reservoir. This makes the penis erect.

The cylinders are deflated by pressing the deflation button for 7 seconds. This transfers fluid back into the reservoir making the penis flaccid. The penis can be made more flaccid by squeezing on the penis shaft.

AMS Ambicor 2-piece Inflatable Penile implant

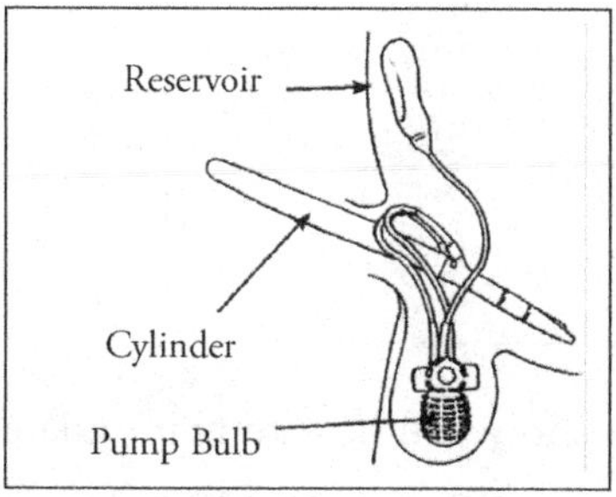

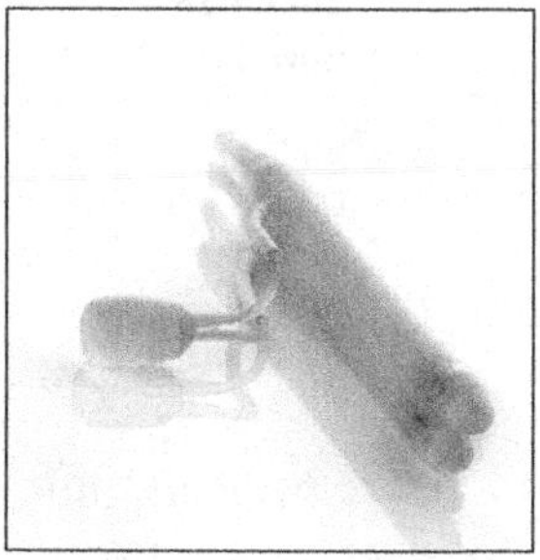

Photos Courtesy of Boston Scientific

Another model that is offered by Boston Scientific is called AMS Ambicor 2-piece Inflatable Penile implant. The AMS Ambicor™ Penile Prosthesis is a closed, fluid-filled system consisting of a pair of cylinders which are implanted in the corpora cavernosa (the penis) and a pump which is implanted in the scrotum. All components are connected by kink-resistant tubing. The device is delivered prefilled with normal saline and preconnected. The cylinders are inflated as fluid is pumped from the reservoirs, which are located in the proximal ends of the cylinders, into the main cylinder body, creating an erection. They are deflated by bending the penis downward causing the fluid to be transferred back to the reservoirs and making the penis flaccid once again.

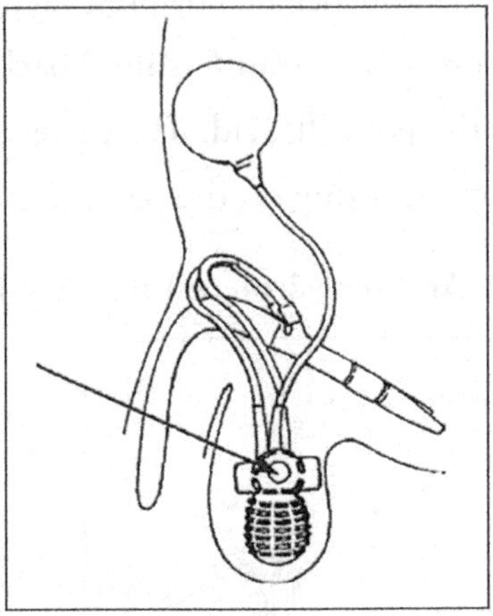

Deflation button

Photos Courtesy of Boston Scientific

Here are some graphics to show you how to manipulate the device to achieve an erection or return to a flaccid state. It looks pretty straightforward and easy to use.

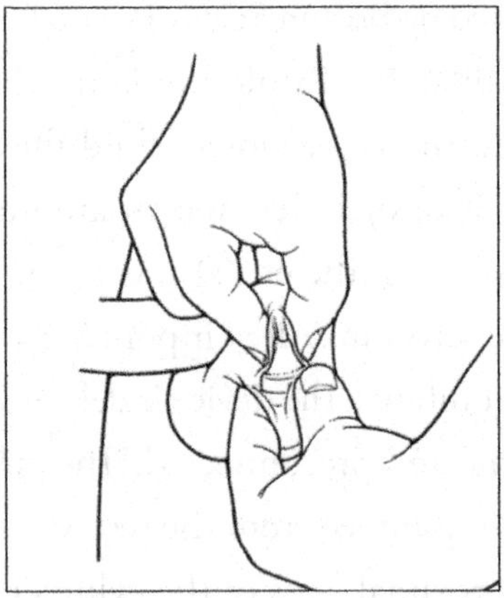

Inflation

Photos Courtesy of Boston Scientific

To inflate the device, squeeze and release the pump bulb several times to make the cylinders stiff. When the cylinders are fully inflated, the pump bulb will be hard and can no longer be compressed.

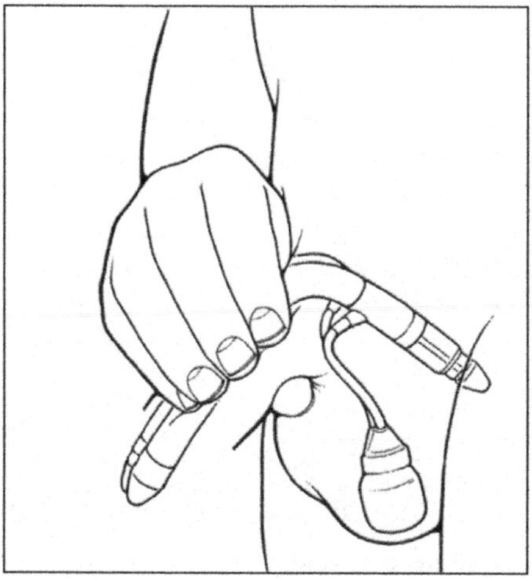

Deflation

Photos Courtesy of Boston Scientific

To deflate the device, the patient places his thumb under the shaft of the penis to act as a fulcrum and his fingers on top of the shaft of the penis. Using the fingers of the same or opposite hand, the patient should bend his penis down over his thumb toward his scrotum to a 55-65-degree angle, making sure that both cylinders are bent. The cylinders should be held in this position for approximately 6-12 seconds and then released. This will open the valves which allow the fluid to flow back into the reservoirs and pump. The patient may also deflate the device by bending the cylinders upwards; this can be done by placing his thumb on top of the shaft of his penis and following the same instructions as above.

- The Tactra™ Penile Prosthesis

Tactra™ Malleable Penile Prosthesis

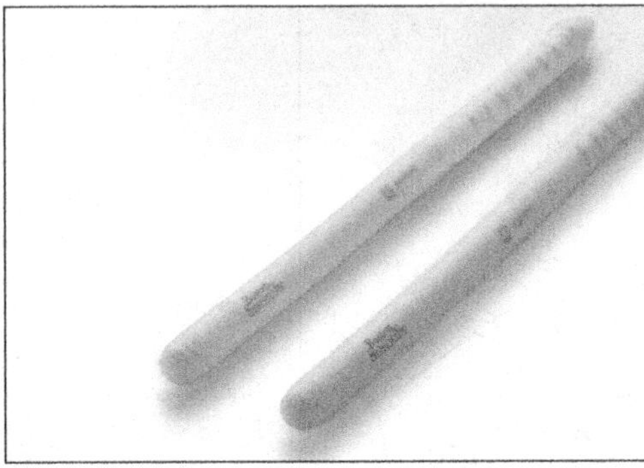

Photo Courtesy of Boston Scientific

Just to make sure that we have almost every man and his personal medical situation covered; I was informed by the Doctor that there is another type of prosthesis that he likes to use in more complicated health situations. This amazing device is straightforward in an effort to accommodate those men who may suffer from conditions like Parkinson's disease, or perhaps even paralysis, where it is difficult to achieve good dexterity with your hands. If your hand is shaking or simply does not move at will, then this option for a penile prosthesis makes it a bit easier for you to enjoy the benefits of a medical device to help with your erections. The Semi Rigid or Malleable Penile Prosthesis is called The Tactra™. The Tactra™ Penile

Prosthesis is designed for enhanced ease of implant for physicians and constructed for durability, offering patients both excellent rigidity and dependable concealment in a device that is natural to the touch.

This prosthesis is rigid at all times, so the patient does not have to manipulate it at all. It is implanted and the penis is always erect. Now this caught my attention completely and I had to ask another question. How does the patient put on his underwear or go around in public without having his erection noticed? The Doctor always has an answer. The Semi Rigid Penile Prosthesis is malleable, and you simply manipulate it to your desired position. I had to stop and think about that for a moment to get a visual in my head of how that actually worked. I immediately thought of bendable toys similar to the Gumby bendable toy.

The Doctor said his patients have been very pleased with the technologies offered for penile prosthesis devices and have told him the devices have been an effective way to get back in the game. When the party is over and it's time to put the device back to a less noticeable position, they easily deflate or bend back to a flaccid position so you can get back to your day-to-day business. With the devices that have saline solution, you can even hurry up the process of deflating the penis by squeezing the penis and pushing the saline solution back up to the reservoir.

Although that may sound painful, it is not and becomes a second way of life with practice.

With the idea of a reservoir inside the man's body as part of several models of penile prosthesis, I wanted to know how often you had to fill up the reservoir due to evaporation of the saline solution. Evidently, according to the Doctor, you only need to fill up the reservoir one time and the device is good for about 10 years. Think of it as similar to a breast implant where the reservoir is made from silicone, filled with saline solution, and is very hardy. We all have an idea of how much manipulation occurs with breast implants, so now just apply that same thought process to the penile prosthesis. That is what makes this book so fun!

After some more thought and starting to understand that penile prostheses were similar to breast implants, due to some of the materials used, I had another question for the Doctor. Does the saline solution from the reservoir models ever leak? If so, how would you know that your penile prosthesis reservoir is leaking since it is inside your body? The answer is that it is also possible as it uses materials similar to a breast implant. However, with a penile prosthesis, the leaks most often occur in the tubing. It's as easy to identify as a flat breast implant because when you try to pump up your prosthesis and you hear "air," you might as well quote Astronaut Jim Lovell who said, "Uh, Houston, we've had a problem."

You will know when it is broken, and at this point, it is time to call your urologist because the penile prosthesis will have to be taken out and replaced. With this predicament and expense, I wondered if these devices have a warranty like a good set of tires. Yes, they do! These devices are covered for the first year. My advice to all recipients of these outstanding devices is to use them as much as humanly possible the first year and get your money's worth and mileage on all the parts before they go out of warranty.

When the Doctor does an inflatable prosthesis for his patients, his number one request is for "a bigger one." Everybody reading this book right now wants to know if this is possible. Society almost demands that a man's penis be as large as possible. I have never really understood this social norm until I dated a guy that had the tiniest penis I have ever seen outside of my days of babysitting infants. I knew right away that the infantile-size penis was not going to work no matter how clever he tried to be. That's another story all together so we will keep moving right along.

The Doctor enlightened me by saying that not one single man is satisfied with his size. So, I asked another very important question. Do you make their penises bigger? The Doctor has crafted this answer for all of his patients in a brilliant way by telling them this: "I can only give you what God already gave you. I am not better than he is. I can make it functional, but your size will remain the same, and I promise it will be functional." He assured me that not one patient has questioned that answer, and all have been pleased with his response.

As a wife, it would seem to me that the only thing that would matter in this discussion would be the fact that an erection can be achieved. But I am not denying that curiosity does creep in and I begin to wonder how big he could make this new penis! This created yet another question for the Doctor. What size are the implants? Of course, the doctor gives me the measurements in metric. So I ask for a more visual idea. If you were to compare the penile implant to a bullet, would it be like a 50 caliber? The Doctor said it is not possible to compare penile prosthesis to bullet calibers. What do I know about bullets anyways? So, I asked another question about the youngest and oldest patients he had used these devices on. I asked this to see how big of a net we could cast so men are aware that they have options. The Doctor's youngest patient for a penile prosthesis was in his 30s and his oldest patient was in his 90s. The surgeries were done after all pre-surgical clearances were met. Both patients were very happy.

When a man has not been able to have sex, and then he can start having sex again, the Doctor reported that his patients are the happiest men on earth. I can assure you these devices do work. How do I know? Well first, not all penile prosthesis patients with the Semi Rigid device are experts at putting that weapon down properly. The Doctor assured me that this skill improves with practice. We can be sitting at any restaurant in our small town or attend any event in town, and inevitably, one of his patients will show up and give the doctor a big hardy handshake and then a hug and always with a huge smile. This is my cue to walk away quickly and find something else to do because the conversation is going straight to the penis. If I am not able to escape, I focus very intently on the surrounding artwork in the room in an effort to divert my eyes from the recipient of a penile prosthesis. This is an industry hazard in our circle of acquaintances when we are out in public. The patient will proceed to discuss how an erection has been achieved. Next, the index finger will come out and the patient will often show the angle or degree of achieved erection with a giant smile on his face. By the way, they never approach the doctor with their wife. I have not figured this out yet. The wife is probably as shy as I am about the subject, since she is the intended target of this newly achieved erection.

So, gentlemen, you are not alone with this issue. The Doctor has heard so many stories over the years from thousands of his patients, both male and female, of how urological problems affect relationships both positively and negatively. The Doctor would encourage you to get to your urologist immediately and seek assistance to improve your quality of life. And this includes young (and older) men who have diabetes or high blood pressure. Surprisingly, these issues can affect your sex life and relationships and you should seek out a qualified urologist immediately in an effort to reduce the emotional suffering that can occur.

Chapter 10

DIABETES AND ERECTILE DYSFUNCTION

Be well and be free

Being the Doctor's wife, I had to ask why on earth would diabetes affect erections. After all, isn't diabetes caused by blood sugar problems? I was not making the connection between blood sugar and erections. Evidently, there is a huge connection between the two and it's because diabetes blocks the arteries which are much smaller in the penis. Therefore, the penis is usually the first piece of real estate that is affected by the shutdown of blood flow. With this understanding, it's easier to understand why this category has increased over time and is more prevalent in certain demographics of the young male, who was diagnosed with diabetes when he was a child or a teenager.

I realized in all my years as the Doctor's wife, I've never been approached by a mom who was concerned about her young son's potential for erectile dysfunction. It dawned on me that moms are not usually thinking that far ahead.

If we were to start educating parents about the effects of diet and obesity and how it will affect their son's life down the road with regards to his ability to perform, I bet it would get the attention of the dads. And it could potentially create a movement strong enough to address juvenile diabetes and its effects on sexual function as an adult.

So, let's get a quick lesson on the two types of diabetes so the concept of blood sugar and blood flow help you understand why erectile dysfunction presents in diabetics. There is Type 1 and Type 2 diabetes. Type 1 diabetics are at the highest risk for impotence because they often have related complications such as kidney failure and heart disease. Since Type 1 diabetes starts at such a young age, these men may have a higher incidence of erectile dysfunction. In general, the longer the patient has had diabetes, the higher the risk for erectile dysfunction. It is even more common for these young diabetic men to lose their partners over this issue and that is what prompts them to seek treatment. Type 1 diabetes is a tragic health issue for boys who became diabetic when they were a child or teenager because, as the Doctor has observed in his 25 years of practice, these young ones may be completely impotent by their 20s or 30s.

When these young patients come in, or with any man suffering from erectile dysfunction, they often do not understand that it may be an underlying health issue that is causing the dysfunction. Most men will blame themselves or have frustration and anger about not being able to perform. They don't realize that erectile dysfunction has nothing to do with them but is related to their health history. The Doctor always makes it a point to tell his patients that he has never seen a male diabetic patient that does not develop erectile dysfunction at some point in his lifetime. According to the Doctor's observations and experience, there is nothing outside of an inflatable penile prosthesis that can help them at some point, which is a good solution to a challenging health history.

Type 2 diabetics are not safe from erectile dysfunction either. Apparently, the longer diabetes is present, it may be an indicator that erectile dysfunction will develop. Let's say that you are 35 years old and you have now developed Type 2 diabetes. You may also start to show symptoms of erectile dysfunction. In addition, diabetes and erectile dysfunction in younger men are now recognized as obvious markers used to evaluate a potential future cardiac event. According to the Doctor, it is very important to let your primary care doctor know that you are starting to experience difficulty with your erections and then he or she can check your cholesterol and blood work and get you started on the necessary medications and healthy lifestyle choices. Ask your primary care doctor to start monitoring you for high blood pressure and cholesterol and follow their instructions to keep these things under control. With these steps, erectile dysfunction can be mitigated if you continue to follow up with your doctor and their advice.

Chapter 11

IS IT COLD OUTSIDE OR ARE THEY ACTUALLY SHRINKING?

Illusions are only in the mind

Well, if it isn't one thing, it's another. You have possibly already been adversely affected to some degree by erectile dysfunction and your mind started playing out every bad scenario you could possibly think of. However, during your thought process, you became incredibly fatigued and wondered why the heck you were so darn tired in the middle of a great day. Or even worse, you have absolutely no desire to have sex.

Turns out you could be one of the many men who are suffering from shrinking testicles or what the Doctor would technically describe as "Low testosterone." These are the recurring advertisements you see on TV where they nicknamed it "Low T." That's the cool way to say that your libido is shot. In the Doctor's opinion, there is an epidemic of Low "T" among men. He sees an average of 10 men each week who come into see him because they have zero desire to get laid. This affects age groups generally from the 30s and older.

It seems that the general population is a bit more educated about lack of desire because of commercials like the one with Frank Thomas, the famous baseball player, who shares his thoughts about a natural wonder drug to improve this situation.

Low T can occur as young as your 30s, but much more in your 50's. Your body will let you know if you are willing to listen and that is your opportunity to fix it. When it comes to testosterone products, you lucky guys will be happy to know that you can benefit from not only an erection that could carry your suitcase, but an improved metabolism, a healthier heart, and better brain function. You will be as sharp as a warrior on the battlefield and ready to take on the world. Sounds too good to be true, but it is actually true.

The American Sexual Society of North America and the American Urological Society recommend a range of testosterone levels to be somewhere between 300 and 950. It is recommended to restore your testosterone levels to a normal range with 400 to 500 being optimal. This optimal range will solve your energy levels, metabolism problems, and general overall sense of well-being. Testosterone has been shown to increase mental acuity, concentration, sense of well-being, and happiness.

You can relax a little bit and stop panicking over the fact that you may need a penile implant. However, you will need to get to your urologist so the doctor can check your testosterone levels by doing a simple blood test. Now, I know you think you can go to your family practice doctor and get the same thing done. However, remember that a urologist is trained to not only look at the results of your testosterone level, but is also trained to ask very specific questions and rule out other potential male problems. I'm sure your imagination is taking off right about now as to what those other problems could be and that is why you go to a urologist instead of a family practice doctor for this particular issue.

There are several symptoms with Low T, and they can be as simple as being a grumpy old man to as terrifying as erectile dysfunction. Testosterone is a very important hormone for men, and when it is out of whack, it's just not as fun to spank the monkey anymore. As a matter of fact, low testosterone levels can even diminish penis sensation and make it even harder to achieve the victory lap of the coveted orgasm. Now if you are wondering why you have had a dramatic reduction in ejaculation, Low T may be the culprit. It's just so much more impressive to leave behind the mother lode and it confirms your manhood and virility as far as society is concerned. When you notice these slight changes, you can relax a little bit because the Doctor exists for a reason. To fix your penis.

I have heard the doctor discuss this subject ad nauseam. But I have also been on the receiving end of Low T and would now consider myself an expert wife on the subject. I can attest to many of the symptoms as demonstrated by the doctor. I am super sure I will be very unpopular with him for revealing this, but the purpose of over sharing is to let readers know that the Doctor is dealing with the same thing you are.

I noticed that the Doctor had become a little bit grumpy and fatigued. I also noticed that he had some difficulty maintaining an erection. Now as the hot wife, I was sure that my hotness had diminished in some way and was adversely affecting our date night. This went on for some time and obviously created some tricky obstacles in our marriage. Because I was married to "The Doctor," I could not believe that we were having these issues. This was only supposed to happen to his patients. Now remember, I am not a doctor, so I had no idea what to do. I didn't even bring up the subject. I pretended that the doctor was still the hottest man on earth and tried to ignore his frustration and stress with this new situation. I knew the doctor had the solution somewhere in that textbook brain of his. I was counting on it.

As time went on, I started to think that it was his blood pressure pills as he was changing medication in an effort to keep it under control. Time continued forward, and suddenly, I heard a new sound in the bathroom every morning. It was a mysterious sound as if he was playing with some kind of toy. It was every single morning. I soon learned the Doctor had embarked upon a pharmaceutical approach to his Low T problem. As time went on, those strange two clicks every morning were the greatest sounds I ever heard.

I learned he was now applying a compounded version of testosterone cream. I began to notice several awesome changes with the doctor. The best change initially was the fact that he was less grumpy. A grumpy man is just not sexy. If you want to get laid, gentlemen, you cannot be grumpy. I then noticed that the Doctor had more energy. This combination of not being grumpy and having more energy got us back to a point where everything else was manageable and a little more positive. The next great thing that unfolded as the morning clicks continued was the fact that date night was back to a point where my man was rocking it and making marriage fun again. I knew he was feeling good again because he would wake up in the morning feeling like a king.

I can now attest that Low T, or more technically correct, "Hypogonadism," can and does significantly reduce the quality of life for men and their partners. I watched it happen to the Doctor. Luckily, he was highly educated and trained on the subject and found a solution before it started to cause further problems at home.

In addition to your marriage, Low T can also have a negative impact on your job. This is because it's difficult to show up for work every day when you are constantly fatigued and irritable.

So now that you are wise to the two click magic cream, it's good to know there are more options you can discuss with your urologist. Testosterone can be delivered to your body in several ways including through cream, transdermal patch, topical gel, tablets, implanted pellet, or injections. There is so much of this stuff on the market, and only available through your doctor, that there is no reason to suffer any longer. Each method of delivery works and is chosen mainly due to insurance coverage. And each method has pros and cons but the only thing that really matters is your dosage. You do need to check your levels the first month to check if they have normalized and to adjust the dose appropriately, and then every six months after that. This is mandatory!

These follow-up appointments are very important because testosterone therapy may have side effects. By monitoring your levels every six months, your urologist can check your PSA (Prostate-Specific Antigen), blood volumes, and testosterone levels to ensure that all is well.

Because I am married to the Doctor, my dad was the lucky recipient of excellent medical care with regards to his Low T. The doctor checked my dad out and decided he was fatigued and mentally foggy due to Low T. The Doctor was correct. My dad's testosterone was at 178 which explained everything.

My dad immediately started the two click magic cream, and within a month, he was coming back to life. He went back for a blood test and he scored a perfect 325. The Doctor sent my dad home to continue with his golf game and life with my mom. About five months later, my mom started telling me that my dad was being very snappy and grumpy, and she wondered if he was either getting dementia or starting to have little strokes. I had wondered the same thing. My dad is about the nicest man on earth. He's a very happy, jovial Irish guy, who only has nice things to say to everyone. This new cranky behavior was certainly out of character for him.

One day, our wonderful gardener, Moses, had come by my dad's house to do his usual job. Moses loved my parents and always watched over them and their beautiful yard. On this unusual day, Moses called me and was quite distressed on the phone. He told me that he was sure my dad was having a stroke. I asked him what made him think this. Moses told me that just after he finished blowing the front walkway, my dad came out the front door and told Moses that he missed a piece of "paper" and to "pick this sh*t up." Now this is absolutely not how my dad behaves. When Moses told me this, I too was sure that my dad was having a minor stroke. I immediately called the doctor and told him what was going on. The doctor started to chuckle. I asked him what was so funny. He said to bring my dad into his office so he could check his testosterone levels with a quick blood test. My dad's testosterone level was 1,028! Holy crap!

I asked the Doctor what he had done to my dad and why his levels were so high. He told me that a small percentage of patients will over absorb the testosterone. It turns out that our family is "drug sensitive" and we do tend to overdose more easily than the average person. So we only use about a quarter of the dosage of the average person. My dad was taken off the testosterone for about two weeks and his dosage was readjusted for his body. My dad is 91 today and continues with the two click magic cream and still plays 18 holes of golf about four days a week.

Chapter 12

THE PROSTATE, A.K.A., THE TRICKSTER

Strength is an understated value

The prostate is an interesting subject, and although most men will smile or laugh along with "pee" jokes, deep down inside, they are harboring a deep-seated fear that they never discuss with anyone. According to the Doctor, by the time a male patient arrives in his office, he is no longer laughing, and the last thing he wants to hear is a pee joke. This is not a voluntary trip and the last thing he wants to talk about is his prostate.

Most people don't know what the prostate is actually for and how it may interfere with a man's ability to pee. The prostate is a walnut-sized gland at the base of a man's bladder. It surrounds the urethra, which is the tube that connects your bladder to your pee hole allowing your pee to exit in fine fashion. The prostate's main purpose is to produce a fluid that transports a man's sperm during ejaculation ensuring a perfect delivery every time. Now imagine if the prostate surrounding the urethra gets bigger and bigger and essentially chokes off the urethra. Peeing becomes a magic act and you realize it's time to get to a urologist.

When a man gets to this point, he is having so much difficulty peeing or emptying his bladder, he is convinced it must be the start of prostate cancer. This is why it takes men so long to make that appointment with the urologist. Not only is it embarrassing and humiliating to describe how your pee stream sounds like skipping rocks on a lake, or that you feel like you are never able to empty your bladder, but the possibility of prostate cancer lies beneath this entire conversation.

Now just to start this conversation off properly with regards to all things "prostate," let's be very clear about what I will call "The Little Trickster." I call it this because the Doctor said there are ZERO symptoms for prostate cancer, unless it is already in the advanced stages. Did you hear me on that one? There are ZERO symptoms for prostate cancer in the early stages. And, if you have shown up to the urologist with weight loss or bone pain, it's probably too late.

This walnut-sized piece of anatomy that exists in the male body is truly a trickster. I would equate it to that of the unpredictable woman. One minute, she is the thing that confirms you still have your manhood, and the next minute, she has betrayed you and walked off with half your stuff. You didn't even see it coming. It comes at you like a right hook from the heavyweight champion of the world.

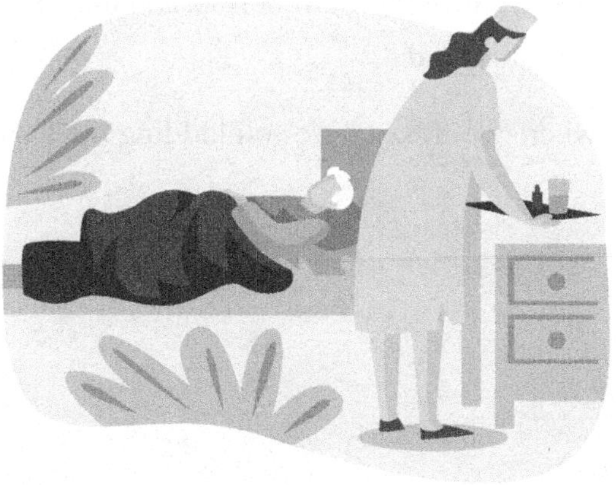

Lower urinary tract symptoms can be one of the very last indicators of prostate cancer and when most men will finally make that appointment. The most common way to diagnose prostate cancer is an isolated elevation of the Prostate-Specific Antigen or PSA. A simple blood test is still a very important part of your urological exam even though it cannot be relied upon solely to determine if you have any issues. Sorry to break the news to all you men out there. While the simple blood test is amazing, it must also be accompanied by the famous digital rectal exam. According to the Doctor, a digital rectal exam is a strong confirmation or denial in most cases of prostate cancer when combined with the PSA. Don't get your hopes up too high just yet. Remember, we are dealing with a trickster. This walnut-sized trickster can go undetected with a normal PSA and a digital rectal exam! That's because PSA is a protein produced by both normal and malignant cells of the prostate gland.

This is where we all say, "Are you kidding me?!"

Chapter 13

THE 3 GENERAL TYPES OF PROSTATE CANCER JUST TO KEEP IT SIMPLE

To try and understand is a beginning

There are essentially 3 types of prostate cancer that are used as a very general guideline. Because this is not a medical book, we are not going to go all "medical science" on you here. After listening to the doctor drown me in his thoughts on the types of prostate cancer, I decided to keep it simple and generalize the topic in a way that was clear for people like me and you. After several sessions at IHOP, while enjoying our pancakes, I felt as though I heard the Doctor say there are generally three categories of bad dudes or groups of cancer to contend with if the prostate, a.k.a. "The Trickster," decides to cause problems.

The three general types are:

1. "Well Differentiated" which is considered to be low-grade and is most likely to be less aggressive and may

tend to grow or spread very slowly. This is often found in older individuals.

2. "Moderately Differentiated" which has features of the well differentiated or the poorly differentiated types. It will behave depending on which of those two features is predominant in the tumor. So, you can have a moderately differentiated tumor that is either slow or fast growing.
3. "Poorly Differentiated" is just plain nasty. This is the one that every man fears and with good reason. Thank goodness it is also the least common type of prostate cancer.

With poorly differentiated cancer, you can have no symptoms and a normal PSA and end up with one of the worst prostate cancers. The reason prostate cancer makes PSA is because the tissue looks like prostate cancer, but just more of it because it multiplies faster and makes more PSA, so it is abnormal. This type of cancer is so bad that it no longer looks like a prostate and the cell is so undifferentiated that it grows like wildfire. It does not make PSA and does not have any features of the prostate, so people think that because their PSA is normal, they don't have prostate cancer. The trickster strikes again. It's for this reason that a digital rectal exam is essential to be done in addition to the PSA.

I have a very good friend, who we shall call Mike for the sake of privacy, who is a smart guy and is hugely involved in his community making the world a better place every day. Mike is a modest guy and is the quiet macho type who would never bother to go to his urologist, let alone submit to a digital rectal exam. The years progressed, and as Mike got older, the more stubborn he became about what he would and would not do. He felt that going to a urologist initially was just too embarrassing. As he neared the age of 65, he started having tremendous difficulty peeing, like every other guy his age.

During Mike's initial visit to find out why it was so hard to pee, the doctor wanted to take the opportunity to check his PSA. This quick blood test revealed that Mike's PSA was 3 and would be considered normal. The range for a normal PSA is 0 to 4. As the appointment continued, Mike was educated by the doctor on the importance of a digital rectal exam and that it was the standard of care for every man his age. Besides that, the doctor was not going to let Mike leave without understanding the risks of not doing it.

I am sure you can guess the rest of the story from here. The digital rectal exam revealed a rock hard prostate, which could have explained Mike's difficulty in peeing. The doctor explained the importance of proceeding with a scheduled prostate biopsy to find out why his prostate was so hard. Sometimes a hard prostate is just that and no further care is needed. Sometimes a rock-hard prostate can be cancer.

When the pathology came back from the lab about a week later, the results showed that Mike indeed had prostate cancer. The Trickster strikes again. According to the Doctor, this can happen as often as 20% of the time in patients.

The size of the prostate, however, is no indication for cancer. The normal size for a prostate is about 25 grams. There are patients who can have a prostate as large as 300 grams with no symptoms whatsoever and still be healthy. Go ahead and do the math on that one. That's a lot of walnuts in there. Obviously, being the wife of the Doctor, I had to ask how on earth does that big thing fit in there? The Doctor assured me that it fits just fine in that particular patient. And evidently, you can have your prostate measured for size if your urologist does an ultrasound.

So, here is the real reason the Trickster is such a problem. It lives up to the nickname I have given it. The prostate can be a normal size and full of cancer with horrible symptoms. Or, you can have a little prostate with no cancer and still have horrible symptoms. Or you can have a prostate that is 300 grams with no symptoms and not have prostate cancer. As usual, size does not matter as in this case. The Trickster can come in all shapes and sizes and either be a good guy or a bad guy with no symptoms or indicators of its status.

You should be reaching for the number of your local board-certified urologist at this point in the book.

When it comes to prostate cancer, there are no two patients alike. There are several ways to treat prostate cancer, which is a discussion to have with your urologist. With treatments like radiation, both external beam radiotherapy and brachytherapy available, surgery may be avoided. If surgery is necessary, there are two ways to remove the prostate, which is either open or robotic surgery. For this very reason, you must be your own best detective and use every tool at your disposal to make sure you stay healthy. Don't wait for prostate cancer to metastasize or spread throughout the body. You have choices to battle this disease if you act early. Depending on the stage of the cancer, your PSA, and how much prostate cancer there is, combined with your age, you have an "optimal" choice for your prostate cancer surgery. You can do radiation or a prostatectomy, and your urologist will discuss all the options that are best for your situation.

Now you know why I call this challenging organ the Trickster. If I say prostate, every man will hear "cancer." The most common solid organ cancer in men is prostate cancer. The prostate has a simple role in the human anatomy and that is to produce the liquid part of the ejaculate along with seminal vesicles that secrete fluid that are partially composed of semen. The Trickster is like the man with a briefcase full of diamonds because it stores the sperm that are ejaculated and sews your seeds for life! Taking out the prostate is difficult both emotionally and physically because it renders you infertile. But you can still have an orgasm, so the party is not completely over yet. Hallelujah!

I did have another question for the Doctor, and it was just idle curiosity. I wanted to know what the youngest and oldest age was of men in which he had to remove the prostate. The youngest guy he operated on was 38 years old. That just broke my heart. Evidently, he had a history of prostate cancer in his family. The oldest was 76.

The average age for dealing with prostate cancer is in your 60s. It can start earlier, depending on your family history or just plain bad luck. The key to dealing with the prostate is to visit your urologist on a regular basis and stay ahead of the game to improve your odds of beating this horrible disease.

So, with all this information, I had to ask the Doctor about the research behind prostate cancer and where we are currently with finding answers to this horrific disease.

If the blood test and symptoms and rectal exam cannot detect prostate cancer, what is being done to solve this health crisis? The Doctor said science is coming up with many approaches to solving this and there are hundreds of millions of dollars being spent in the hope of early identification with this disease.

Free PSA (fPSA) tests are some of the newest approaches to detecting prostate cancer, which is somewhat of a complicated approach, but also has many false negatives. There is another method called PSA velocity, which looks at the rate of rise for the PSA and is done about every six months. You measure the PSA velocity, which is essentially the PSA divided by the prosthetic volume or the size of the prostate, and that has some hope for identifying cancer. There is also a "super sensitive" PSA that is more likely to possibly detect cancer. The verdict is still out on that and is not widely available yet. There is a urine test called a PCA3 that is also available, but not widely used yet. You can ask your urologist which test may be best for you.

There are two common causes for a falsely elevated PSA. The first one is prostatitis where inflammation of the prostate causes PSA to leak out and give you a high PSA result. The second reason for a falsely elevated PSA is if the patient has a PSA done within 30 days of a prostatitis, Foley catheter, or colonoscopy. These items may likely cause the PSA to be abnormal. However, a referral to a urologist for those reasons does not warrant a prostate biopsy. A waiting period of 30 days is warranted to allow the PSA to come back to the level it was prior to the cause of the rise. If it is still high after 30 days, then this would be cause for concern. If it is normal, then no further evaluation is warranted.

Prostatitis is simply an infection of the prostate and is often treated with an antibiotic for four weeks. However, this aggravated condition can cause a man great discomfort and inconvenience due to constant urination, all while wondering if he has prostate cancer.

Remember, the Trickster can be symptomatic or completely cloaked like Harry Potter and symptom free. You just don't know what you are dealing with and so you must leave it to your board-certified urologist to do a PSA and digital rectal exam on a regular basis.

Chapter 14

NO, MEN LEAK, TOO?

Humility is to see reality

So, gentlemen, the ladies have decided to give you equal rights when it comes to peeing your pants. I bet you didn't see this coming! As it turns out, the Trickster in the last chapter is not done yet. The prostate continues to cause problems that can eventually lead to incontinence. For all you men nearing the age of 60, or those lucky enough to make it even further, this chapter is for you.

It's easy to relate to the topic of incontinence when you are simply people watching in a busy location like an airport, waiting for your connecting flight. Just sit and watch the traffic in and out of the men's bathroom in any public location. You will notice that older men heading for the restroom will often pick up the pace as they get closer to the bathroom door. But they try to do it in a way that nobody will actually notice their strides are longer and slightly faster. This human observation is why I decided to write this chapter.

Usually the problem of incontinence or leakage begins when a man stands up and gravity takes over. I notice this with my dad, who is 91and deserves a medal of honor for making it this far. As he stands up, he will start to go do something else, and I will try to talk to him as he's passing by. He happily interrupts me and says gravity is in charge and must cut our conversation short to answer to the porcelain god, a.k.a., "the toilet."

Incontinence is just one symptom but may have many different causes as to why you might leak. There are two main types – stress and urge. Urge incontinence can happen because of overactive bladder, lifestyle choices, age, and without any male surgeries messing up the plumbing. Stress incontinence is usually the result of a male surgery like prostate surgery and is out of your control.

Urge incontinence is when you have the need to pee immediately and often, morning, noon, and night. With this condition, a man will start to plan his day around all the available bathrooms that can be accessed quickly or when the urge hits. Such behavior has been described by the Doctor as bathroom mapping. It's not uncommon for a man to actually pee his pants should he not find a toilet in time.

The possible reasons for urge incontinence can be due to several health conditions such as infection, enlarged prostate, inability to completely empty your bladder, or even issues with your urethra that may actually block your pee hole from allowing urine to exit properly. Let's not forget good old-fashioned overactive bladder (OAB). Age is another possible culprit when it comes to urge incontinence. Once you hit the magic number of about 60, the odds of leaking are in your favor. Another potential reason for urge incontinence can also be psychological stress and diet. These are all the things to consider when you are constantly feeling the urge to pee all day every day. Both urge and stress incontinence interfere with quality of life!

Stress incontinence is a step up from urge incontinence and can actually interfere with your quality of life more so than urge incontinence. Stress incontinence is most common in women but can also happen to men and is out of your control. Your plumbing leaks when it is introduced to any kind of physical exertion. A man may pee his pants every time he sneezes, coughs, laughs, stands, or even lifts, pushes or pulls. These normal human activities that are a part of everyday life make it almost impossible to enjoy a simple day of rest and relaxation or even a day out with the guys. Leaking is not only damn inconvenient, it's simply just not sexy. Be kind to the women in your life who suffer from this condition. It's common in a lot of women.

The biggest reason behind stress incontinence in men is when the prostate gland has to be removed due to prostate cancer. There are other types of urogenital surgery that may cause stress incontinence, which is any surgery to do with your male plumbing. When a urologist has to start messing around with things down there, leakage can begin.

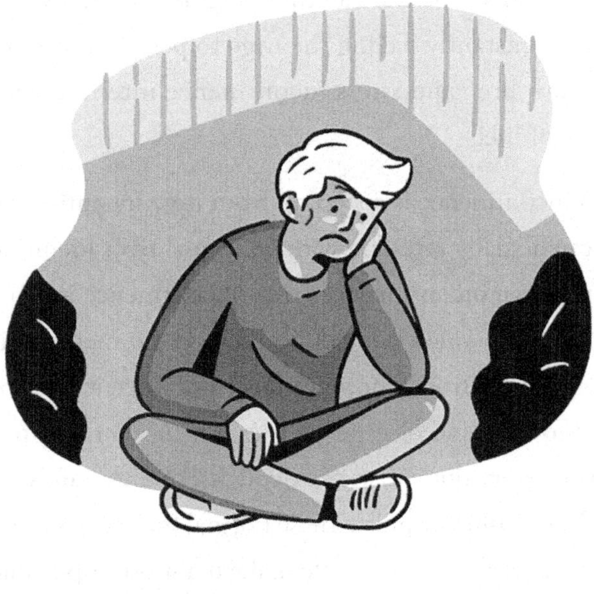

There are treatment options for both urge and stress incontinence. Although the entire subject seems like painful, and it is, and it is, there are great solutions for men. For urge incontinence, you will probably finally get yourself to a urologist when you have hit that breaking point of exhaustion as urge incontinence is the monster that never lets you sleep. This is because it's a 24-hour problem. Pipes don't stop leaking just because you are trying to sleep. If you have stress incontinence, you will get plenty of sleep, but as soon as you wake up and head to the bathroom, you will probably leave a trail of urine on the floor and not even know it. Both forms of incontinence in men require multiple trips to the toilet.

The good news with incontinence in men today is that there are a variety of solutions depending on your type of incontinence and level of severity. These solutions range from diet, bladder training, pelvic floor physical therapy, absorbent pants, medications, and even surgery. A good urologist will work with you to solve your incontinence issues depending on your personal health history and condition.

Regardless of the potential reason behind the constant urge to pee or any kind of leak, it's time to seek out your board-certified urologist and get this issue solved! There are no more reasons to feel depressed or even isolated. A good urologist has a menu of treatments to help you get through this very difficult situation that affects almost 6 million men in the U.S. alone.[1] So be the brave man, you

1 About Incontinence—Contributing Factors—Prostate Problems in Men. The Simon Foundation for Continence. http://www.simonfoundation.org/about_incontinence_contributing_factors_prostate.html. Accessed September 13, 2016.

once were and take the steps to solving your leak. The solutions are good ones and Millions of men are already benefiting from these treatments. Get the help you need to finally get some sleep or stop leaving a trail of urine on the floor and rejoin your family and friends in life.

Chapter 15

PENILE TRACTION. IT WORKS!

Do what you can and persevere

This last year, the Doctor and I attended the annual Sexual Medicine Society of North America meeting, in Nashville, Tennessee. As usual, we arrived at our hotel and went through the check in process to get up to our room after a long day of travel. Not 15 minutes after we arrived, there was a knock at the door. I paused my unpacking to answer the door and was met by one of the hotel bellman. He looked me dead in the eye and quickly handed me some type of trade show flyer. As I looked down to see what the heck it was, I was turning it around and over to realize that it was a replica of a bent cucumber with some writing on it and a "bump". I looked up to try and ask the bellman what the heck this was and immediately realized that he had disappeared down the hallway like a lightning bolt. I re-examined the flyer and realized that it was a flyer to promote penis health and address a common problem known as Peyronie's disease. No wonder the bellman took off so fast. How odd to be handed a cardboard cucumber with a bend and a bump, unless you are at the annual meeting for the Sexual Medicine Society of North America, where these problems are solved.

When you hear the term penile traction, the visual created is of those torture devices used in medieval times where they would put you on a stretching rack and pull your arms and legs in different directions to get you to cooperate. The penile traction device is nothing like "the rack." The penile traction device is used to help treat Peyronie's disease in which the patient suffers from a curvature of the penis with a bump when erect. This curvature can show up over time or sometimes right away. Peyronie's disease can shorten the penis and cause painful erections or even soft erections. This condition requires you to get to your urologist as soon as possible because this is not a joke.

Now that I have your full attention, you can uncross your legs and continue to read. I learned about Peyronie's disease through an inquiry by one of the moms in the high school parking lot after parent teacher conferences. This woman came up to me looking around as she approached. Clearly, she was on the down low to try and get some help from the Doctor. When she finally reached me at my car, she was obviously not only perplexed as to how to start this conversation, but clearly quite distressed.

They say that hindsight is 20/20 and now I know why. The subject of a curved penis that is painful and interfering with your sex life is not an easy subject to broach in the high school parking lot. After learning about Peyronie's disease from the Doctor, I now know why this woman seemed stressed. Her husband's pain and panic during an erection and attempt at sex was very real for her and she was determined to find a way to fix it.

As this high school mom started to explain to me the problems with her husband's penis, I knew I needed to remain calm. She described how his erections not only bent upwards, but almost backwards. I caught myself slightly wincing at the description and asked her if he had pain with that angle. She confirmed a high degree of pain and went on to describe that his penis was like a backwards fishhook. It went straight up and then bent backwards toward his belly button.

With all this information from a complete stranger, who I had previously only seen at school gatherings, I found the courage to ask a question that I wanted answered for my own curiosity. I asked her how she got it in. She said it wasn't fitting in anymore and that was the problem. As I was processing all the information this lady was telling me, I was trying to figure out how the heck I was going to relay this unusual problem to the doctor. I needed more information from her. For the next 20 minutes, we discussed her husband's penis behavior for the last year and the types of erections he was getting and when exactly they started to curve in a direction that rendered his penis painful and useless. What a conversation!

I called the Doctor from my car phone and told him that I had something serious to discuss and that it was a bit unusual. I explained the problem as it was relayed to me. When I was done, he named the disease and said it was actually very painful initially. He told me to have this lady get her husband to come into his office in the morning so he could help him. "You've seen this before?" I blurted out. "Of course," he answered. "I'm a urologist. I deal with this on a regular basis."

I hung up the phone with the Doctor and thought long and hard about his response to this man's curved penis problem. I had no idea that the Doctor was dealing with curved penises. This cast a whole new light on the Doctor. I was learning so many strange things about the man I thought I knew so well. Then I wondered why the heck this lady's husband's penis is now part of my reality and how on earth will I ever look at her or him the same the next time I see them out in public.

The treatment for Peyronie's disease is effective and includes injections with or without penile traction devices and/or surgical procedures. When Peyronie's disease presents with erectile dysfunction, the treatment is a penile prosthesis.

I realized my life with the Doctor had made me a part of people's lives in the most intimate way. I never really signed up for this. I just wanted to be an awesome wife and mother, not the assistant coach of the "penis team."

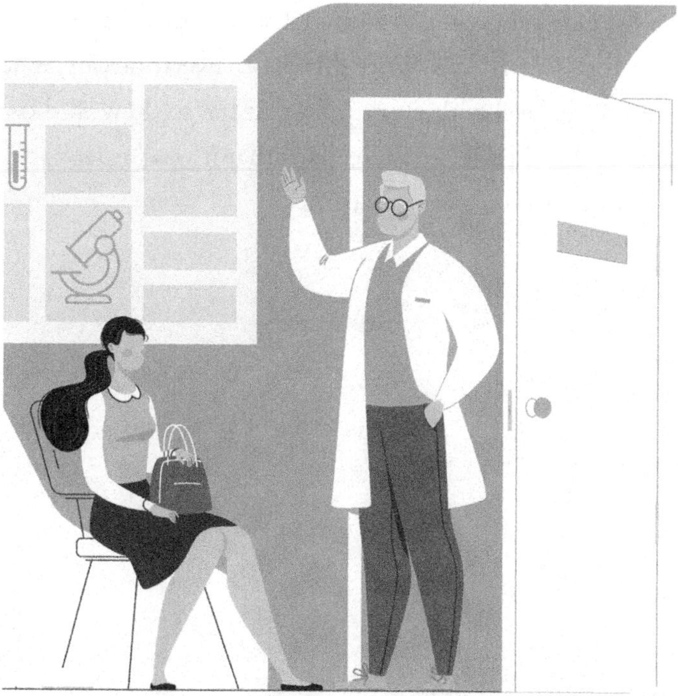

This role as the Doctor's wife was taking a lot out of me in ways I could have never imagined. I had to rely upon my experience of using discretion and kindness for every urology crisis that showed up on my phone, at my table, at my kids' school, in the grocery store, at the spa, on the golf course, or at the airport.

After listening to so many people and their urological problems at every age and stage, I knew I was on to something that truly mattered for people. Urology and quality of life are synonymous with each other. This is one of the reasons I decided to write this book. Everyone can relate on some level with everything that has to do with those parts down there. I also realized that it was just a matter of time before it was my turn.

Chapter 16

LADIES, IT'S YOUR TURN

The Doctor specializes in female pelvic reconstruction

First things First! Let's learn about the difference between your urologist and gynecologist and what the heck a urogynecologist does. You are going to need to understand this information as well as you understand your native language. A urologist deals with anything that has to do with urine. For women, this will include the kidneys, bladder, ureter, and urethra. A gynecologist deals with the reproductive organs, which include the ovaries, uterus, fallopian tubes, cervix, and vagina. Often a gynecologist and urologist will do surgeries together and "hand off" when they have entered the other physicians territory of specialty. A urogynecologist and female pelvic medicine reconstructive urologist are trained to handle both sets of organs. They specialize in Female Pelvic Medicine and Reconstructive Surgery. This is considered a subspecialty of Urology and Gynecology and focuses on the care of women with pelvic floor problems.

Urogynecologists and Female Pelvic Reconstructive Urologists have gone through extensive extra training after completion of residency to be specialized in the diagnosis and management of female pelvic disorders, which may include incontinence, pelvic organ prolapse, pelvic pain and overactive bladder. It seems that Urogynecologists and Female Pelvic Reconstructive Urologists are not as prevalent as Urologists and Gynecologists, so do your homework to find one.

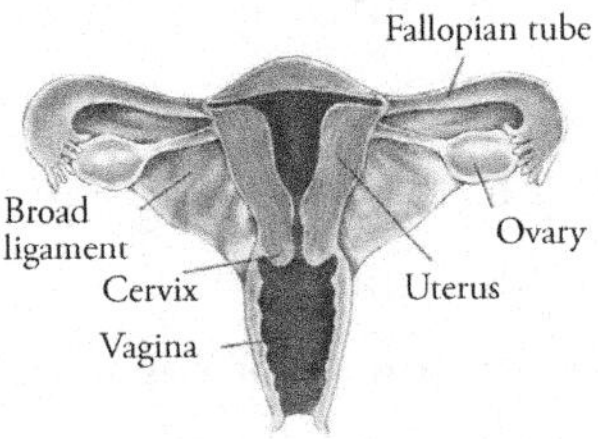

GYNECOLOGIST EXPERTISE
Reference: http://www.aboutcancer.com/gyn_cancer1_normal.htm

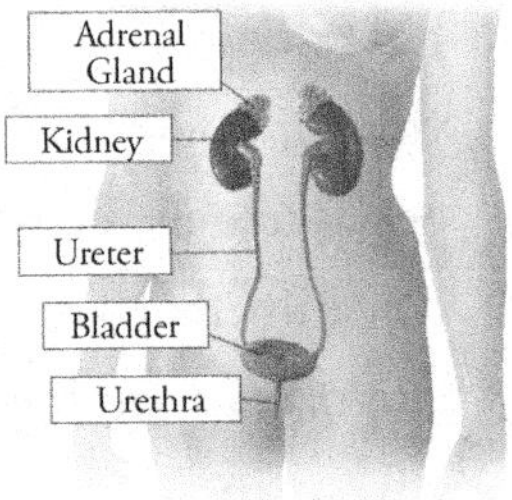

UROLOGIST EXPERTISE
Reference: https://www.mountnittany.org/articles/healthsheets/318

Urogynecologist & Female Pelvic Reconstructive Urologist DO BOTH

So what on earth would the Doctor have to say to us ladies? When I first met the doctor, I had no idea what he did, other than work in the Army. On our second date at Starbucks, I asked him what he did. He told me he was a urologist. I asked, "what's a urologist?" He gave me the most technical and anatomical description I had ever heard in my life, where he even used words such as ureter, prostate, pelvic floor, and incontinence. To sum it up, he said he treats anything that has to do with urine. I thought for a moment as I tried to digest what I had just heard and, in my mind, I determined that he was a plumber. He said he'd never been called a plumber, but that's essentially what he fixed. "It's official, you're a plumber," I said. From that day forward, when anyone has asked me what the doctor does for a living, I simply say he is a plumber. I do this for two reasons. One, it's not important what he does, and two, being married to a urologist is just embarrassing for me personally as I have no interest in openly discussing penises and vaginas.

As the years have passed being married to my "plumber," I have heard every single phone call in the middle of the night when he was on call and even when he was not. Both of our phones ring several times a day from people who need a plumber. Because the subject matter is such uncharted territory for most everyone, and incredibly embarrassing, the wife is often the scout on a mission to find out how to fix the marital plumbing issues for the couple. These scouting missions are for the women's plumbing at least half the time.

The Doctor has informed me that at least 60% of his practice is for treating women. You can imagine my shock the first time I heard this. When I first learned that he treated women, I said, "I thought you were a urologist." He confirmed that he was. I then was foolish enough to ask the second question. "What do women need from a urologist?" The doctor got this big silly grin on his face as though I had just handed over the microphone and he was about to go on stage. He was going to now be able to pontificate about his favorite part of his specialty without any boundaries or rules because I had asked the question. I panicked as I realized my mistake and reached for something to fidget with to try and hide my modesty during another lecture on the human body. The worst part about his lecture was that I was going to hear the word vagina several times and that had everything to do with me and my plumbing.

Chapter 17

LEAKING: FROM DRIP DRIP TO THE RIVER NILE

Don't quit for effort matters

The first reason a woman might end up in the office of a urologist is usually because there has been significant evidence of incontinence, or simply put, peeing your pants. All this time, I did not even know that women leaked. Holy crap, old age was really starting to scare me. Now every woman knows that a little bit of tinkle is absolutely not enough to drag her into the office of an unknown entity called a urologist or whatever the heck it's called. It is simply traumatic to think that one more person is going to look up there for anything other than a baby or the purpose of not making a baby. This was the breadth of my knowledge early in my marriage to the Doctor. I really had no interest as to how the human body worked as a younger woman.

Being with the Doctor for so many years, though, I have come to understand a wide variety of situations that will aggravate incontinence and truly affect the quality of life for a woman. With incontinence, a woman will literally spend her day planning out where all the bathrooms are just in case. Remember, we called this "bathroom mapping" in the male incontinence chapter. This is not only aggravating, but it becomes not worth it to go out and do the things you love.

A woman can experience incontinence and be required to use an excessive number of pads and even go as far as having to change her clothes because they get wet from leakage. They also fear smelling of urine or having a leak at any given moment due to laughing, sneezing, or coughing. A woman may also have to stop certain activities such as working out or physical activities due to leaking while exerting herself.

Younger women are not excluded from incontinence. The number one reason for the younger woman to seek out a urologist is because they may leak urine during sex. It often happens for years and may just be a slight amount in the beginning. Over time, it starts to interfere with sex, and when an orgasm occurs, there is more involved than one would like to mention. This shift in the severity of incontinence is what gets the younger women to seek help.

I have been secretly taking mental notes over the years as I have listened to the Doctor on the phone with the hospital or to the nurses or to his staff. There have been several times when I have left the room because I just didn't want to know any more information about how my body was going to slowly fall apart as the years marched on.

Speaking of the years marching on, that is a perfect Segue to the second top reason women must go and see a urologist. It's called pelvic prolapse. This term initially was like listening to pig Latin the first time I heard it. It seemed like so many syllables and yet, I knew deep down that the doctor was talking about my body. I was almost too afraid to inquire, but because I never seem to learn about asking questions, I of course, proceeded to ask, "What the heck is that?".

The plumber described several body parts that were totally misaligned and hanging by a thread. Well, that's what I thought I heard as those words of Pig Latin were being spoken to me. All I could imagine was that I would have no idea what to do when this happens to me. This problem alone has helped me to see the value in a guy like the doctor, also known as a plumber/contractor.

Evidently, pelvic prolapse is a condition that does affect many women at some point in their life. It can happen as young as your thirties or as late as your 80's, depending on many factors like age, health, number of pregnancies and types of delivery, obesity, and good old DNA. Pelvic prolapse can occur when the tissues and muscles down there, basically run out of muscle power to hold up and in, your uterus, bladder, or even your rectum. For those of you who have had babies, you completely understand what the heck I'm talking about. Here's the part I didn't know. Evidently when the pelvic muscle becomes so weak these organs can come right out of your vagina. Yes, you heard me right. Houston, we have a problem!

Chapter 18

PELVIC PROLAPSE AND YOU STILL WANT TO HAVE SEX?

Challenges are opportunities to keep trying

Pelvic prolapse is a term that very few people have ever heard. The first time I heard the doctor talk about it, he told me it was one of the most severe cases of pelvic prolapse he had ever seen. I was instantly curious about what the hell he was talking about, and once again, I had to ask a urological question that always seems to light the doctor up like a Christmas tree. Urological questions to him are like foreplay on a hot Friday night date with his sexy wife.

My curiosity was piqued, but I was also completely terrified I was going to learn something that could actually happen to me. I knew the doctor was going to lay this out for me like a patient on the table and that to me was like watching the Doctor sew my finger back on.

He began by describing exactly what the pelvic floor is. This is not the nightclub dance floor where you go out and show off your bump and grind. The pelvic floor is actually comprised of the muscles and tissues just below the bladder. Yep, it's another item "up there." These are the tissues that act as the Great Wall of China for your uterus and bladder while having sex.

The pelvic floor acts as a cradle to hold the uterus and bladder in place so they do not sink down into the vagina and interrupt life and cause problems with urine flow. If this happens, you can imagine how the pipes can get bent and convoluted in a way that it can become near next to impossible to pee properly without becoming an acrobat on the toilet. Only the women with pelvic prolapse will slightly chuckle at the visual that popped in their head when they heard the term, toilet acrobat.

Pelvic prolapse occurs when the tissues become weakened and stretch out further than a dried-out rubber band. This concept of the pelvic floor failing or sagging, and no longer able to hold up the bladder and other things nearby, is not such a mystery when you liken it to the overused rubber band that has been stretched out around a stack of files for years and becomes unsuccessful at holding the stack together any longer. The pelvic floor tissue in many women is almost the same. Childbirth certainly does not help a woman, as the pelvic floor gets stretched in ways that men and women alike don't care to think about.

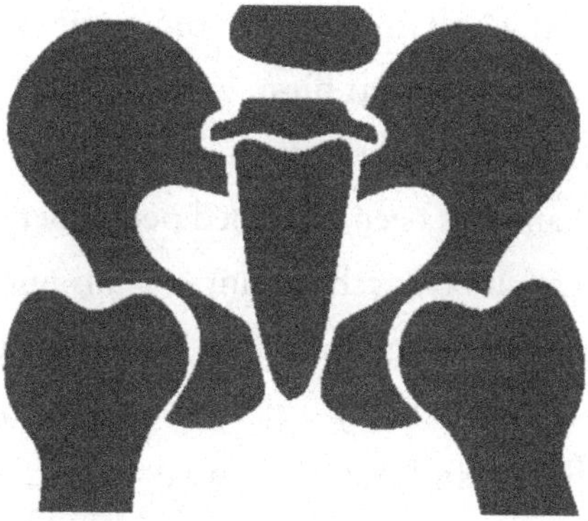

Now that you see how the pelvic floor tissue can stretch out and become weak, where is the pelvic floor muscle actually located? This is a muscle that is attached and stretched from your coccyx, or tailbone, in the back to your pelvic bone in the front. It's similar to an internal diaper or a hammock. I like the second description best. The tissue in the pelvic floor is incredibly delicate, yet highly functional. This is why you want ONLY a board-certified reconstructive urologist, or urogynecologist doing any kind of surgery on you in this area.

It takes years of specific training to fix prolapse and incontinence conditions. The tissue or pelvic floor muscle is essentially the barrier for the organs on the other side. When it weakens or fails, you have a critical situation that alters your quality of life. You are plumbed in a very precise way that allows all urine to exit in an orderly fashion. For the ladies, don't forget that your uterus is up there, too, and we all know what comes out of the uterus every month if you haven't hit menopause yet. That magic little sack that holds life needs a proper way to drain and refresh itself and has been plumbed perfectly to do a very fine job. It's an amazing thing until it falls out into your vagina. Don't let your gynecologist tell you that he or she can fix that. They probably just want your money instead of your wellness, and now you are educated enough to know the difference.

The actual term for when your uterus or possibly even your bladder fall out into the vagina is technically called Pelvic Organ Prolapse (POP). After learning this from the doctor, he tells me that in the worst cases, the prolapsed uterus or bladder can be seen when looking up there or even drop down through the opening of the vagina.

This thought of the uterus or even the bladder falling out through my vagina had me absolutely floored. Of course, we would be talking about the pelvic floor because this is now my life being married to the Doctor. After some time had passed and I had several years to absorb this terrifying example of gravity while trying to enjoy my state of denial, I had run into one of the doctor's medical assistant's out on the town. We got to talking about my book and when I mentioned that I would be writing about the subject of pelvic prolapse, this medical assistant slightly smirked and said, "oh that should be a good chapter"! Right there, I felt a door open to learning more from this amazing gal who has served on the front lines of penises and vaginas along-side the doctor for 15 years.

I proceeded to dive right in and ask the most direct question that every single person wants to know. How the heck does a woman walk if her uterus and or bladder are hanging between her legs? I wondered if it was like walking with a full water balloon between your legs and how the heck would you keep it from leaking? My mind had the most terrifying visual, only because I realized that this happens to so many women, and I happen to be a woman.

This medical assistant was a great source of front-line information and proceeded to tell me that it was always obvious who was at the clinic for pelvic prolapse because they had on the tightest jeans that money could buy. Those jeans were painted on for a reason. I stopped and thought about that for a long minute. Immediately, I felt horrible about all the times I had judged women in jeans so tight that you could play the drums on their butt cheeks and probably get a great sound to reverberate right back at you. I realized in that moment that my judgment of those tight jeans was very unnecessary and very unkind. Who knew that tight jeans were now considered a medical device? With my newfound knowledge, I realized that I will have to face my karma for those judgments, which I thought were simply funny, but actually cruel. Immediately, I heard another one of the doctor's lectures about the seriousness of all thing's urology.

According to this experienced gal on the front lines, the tight jeans hold the uterus and or bladder inside the vagina so the patient does not have to walk with a "water balloon" between their legs as they walk in front of all the other patients to make it to the exam room where help can be found. When the pants come off in the exam room, all hell breaks loose from organs sliding out of the vagina and urine leaking from the newfound freedom of those free flying organs swinging between a woman's legs. As my mind has to work at understanding what I am hearing the medical assistant explain, I almost liken the free-falling female organs to the closest experience they will ever have to being a man with testicles. Right now, I am so happy to be a woman who does not have to deal with the thought of testicles, a.k.a., uterus and bladder, between my thighs.

As she continued to explain pelvic prolapse in great detail, she shared the story of her first pelvic prolapse patient who came in for an exam because she could not pee. The Doctor tells the medical assistant to put in a catheter for the patient and to empty the bladder. This patient was clearly suffering from misaligned plumbing that caused her bladder to become so full that she required the services of a urologist. This was not the first time this patient had to come in to be catheterized from her prolapse condition.

The Doctor walked out of the exam room and left the medical assistant to do her job. Inserting a catheter is one of the first things a medical assistant learns to do in their training and is considered a very simple procedure. As the medical assistant begins, she feels very confident that she knows exactly where the urethra is, which is the pee hole. Strangely, she cannot see the pee hole because the uterus is outside the vagina blocking her view.

Sitting in the chair at the end of the exam table, she starts flipping through the chart because she did not know what to do and did not want the patient to know. After about 15 minutes of pretending that she knew what do with the catheter, she had to leave the exam room and get the doctor. The Doctor came back into the exam room, put on a pair of gloves and simply pushed the uterus back up inside the woman. The medical assistant was so freaked out at the whole experience that she told herself she was never ever having kids. And she never did! After that pelvic prolapse patient experience, the medical assistant became a pro at shoving the uterus and/or bladder back up into its proper geography and subsequently ended up training all the other medical assistants on how to do it correctly.

I thought about the medical assistant training all the other assistants how to shove the organs back up into their original location and wondered how many patients come in for pelvic prolapse. She simply said “LOTS.” I proceeded to think we have an entire small city full of pelvic prolapsed women all wearing tight jeans and only one doctor in our town who knew how to fix them. This is the part of the book where, if you are considering on becoming a doctor, please consider becoming a pelvic reconstructive urologist. There is an actual board certification for this called Diplomat, Female Pelvic Medicine and Reconstructive Surgery. If you ever need this surgery, please find the doctor with this certification.

According to the Doctor, this type of surgery deals with tissue that is extremely delicate, yet if you have it done by the right doctor the first time, you have an outstanding chance of getting close to becoming normal urologically speaking. This generally depends upon your specific situation. However, your quality of life is sure to return, and you can toss those skintight jeans right out the window.

My mother had to have this same surgery done, as she had eight children. She lived with incontinence for almost 40 years. After her surgery, she had wondered why she did not have the surgery done 40 years prior. I can remember that when we would go out and about for the day, we had to map our way around town by the next bathroom stop. I never really understood what the problem was and assumed my mom was drinking far too much water and coffee. But she was actually dealing with the same problem that almost every childbearing woman must deal with at some point.

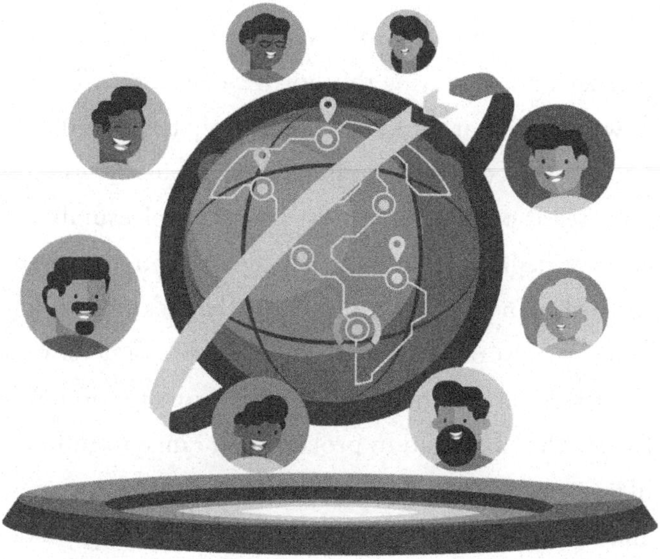

Considering there are almost 7 billion people on the planet, and about half of those are women, it starts to boggle the mind as to why we are not talking about this subject more than we are. I haven't even tapped into the conversation about fistulas where urine simply leaks out as it is made. The point here is that a simple trip to a board-certified urologist trained in pelvic reconstruction is your golden ticket to good urological health. Remember, there are different types of urologists who handle different areas of expertise. After writing this, I used to think I was married to a plumber, but now I'm thinking I might be married to a contractor.

So, let's talk about sex and pelvic prolapse. There are many women who are still having to have sex with their partner while enduring this horrific condition. We have now learned that the organs can simply be pushed back up into the correct geographical location when necessary. Sex is possible, but most likely not pleasurable. If you are beginning to have pain when you are having sex, this can be a good indicator that it's time to get to a urologist or uro-gynecologist. They can determine what kind of treatment is best for your situation. The factors that may lead to prolapse can range from heavy lifting, obesity, and constipation to coughing, sneezing, and laughing too much. Let's not forget about good old fashion estrogen depletion. When your estrogen levels drop and your tissues thin out, the aging process begins, and gravity takes over. Everything starts to head south whether we like it or not.

In addition to hormones and surgery, behavior therapy could also be an option. Imagine my shock when I found out you could do behavior therapy down there. My imagination ran away with all kinds of visuals of my vagina doing weightlifting to water ballet. I was fantasizing about all kinds of activities that would strengthen that pelvic floor muscle.

This brings to my mind a story that another girlfriend came to me with. Everyone knows that I am married to a Doctor who also specializes in vaginas. My childhood girlfriend and I were talking on the phone about incontinence. Turns out that my girlfriend had a remedy in her own mind about what would help stave off incontinence. This dear friend asked if I would run her idea by the doctor to see if it was actually a good solution to incontinence.

I proceeded to listen to my girlfriend with intense curiosity. She tells me that during her 5 mile walks every day up and down the hills of Seattle, she has recently inserted Ben Wa Balls into her vagina during her long walks. She continues to tell me that her entire objective is to keep the balls in place up there, for the entire walk. As she is telling me this, I wondered if she was going to stop somewhere on the hill and simply remove the Ben Wa Balls if they became too much. The visual with this gorgeous woman dropping her spandex pants to pull out her Ben Wa Balls and the exacerbation of relief that would follow was a visual comedy show in my head that I won't soon forget. My first question to her was how many balls she stuck up there. This question alone can clarify whether you are entering a cave or a cavern. My dear friend tells me that she inserts two Ben Wa Balls. I felt a slight relief. I promised her that as soon as the doctor got home from work, I would ask him this very important question.

The Doctor arrived home after a long day from work and I of course am smart enough to know to let him decompress and eat before anything of great importance is discussed. After dinner, I approached with a bit of insecurity and proceeded to tell him that my dear friend called me with a urological question for him. As always, he was happy to listen to his favorite subject.

I explained how my girlfriend was using her Ben Wa Balls in her vagina on her walks. His first question was, "what are Ben Wa Balls"? I was shocked to know that the doctor was unaware of these little gems and started to describe them as steel balls that fit up in the vagina about the size of a ping pong ball. Evidently, they come in different colors, but that is not the point. I told him that she puts them in her vagina and holds them in there as she walks and asked if this had any urological benefits for strengthening the pelvic floor. I was shocked to learn that unless the exact muscles are engaged to hold the balls in place, the exercise is not helpful.

The Doctor tells me that when he is examining a woman and he sticks his fingers in her vagina and asks her to squeeze, most of the time there is absolutely no reaction in the vagina. Evidently, most women will squeeze their butt muscles or belly muscles. The vagina remains unresponsive. The Doctor continued to inform me that unless the patient learns how to identify the vaginal muscles and then can squeeze those specific muscles, no benefit will be gained to help strengthen the pelvic floor. Imagine my shock to learn that a woman cannot squeeze her vagina upon command. Every woman is sure they are squeezing something down there and must be as shocked as me to find out that it only works if you squeeze the right part. If you are so inclined to do so, go ahead and use your own fingers up there and see if you can squeeze your fingers and not your belly muscles or buttocks. That should give you another clue that you may need to schedule an appointment with your urologist.

Now you know some of the most prevalent urological problems for women, incontinence, and pelvic prolapse. These conditions should only be treated by a board-certified urologist who is current in their training and understanding of the newest and most effective ways to take care of your urological health. There are great solutions for these issues to improve your quality of life quickly. The Doctor tells me that a woman waits an average of five years to seek help from a urologist. Women are used to dealing with discomfort and often don't make the time to care for themselves properly until it becomes a crisis, like peeing during an orgasm. Your quality of life is waiting for you to grab the phone and call your board-certified urologist.

Chapter 19

LACK OF DESIRE – WHERE THE HELL IS MY WINE?

To try is courageous

Now ladies, I am sure that most of you know where this is going to go, so let me start by sharing with you the top reason a woman would go see the doctor, the urologist, or the "plumber". It seems that a woman would need to seek out a urologist and not a gynecologist, unless he or she is a urogynecologist because of "lack of desire."

To put it a more directly, you have zero interest in any form of sex, which seems like way too much effort for something with zero return as far as you are concerned. It is just one more person asking for one more thing. Here, all this time, you just thought you were sick and tired of doing everything for everyone. As it turns out, this lack of desire thing is not just exhaustion or too much wine (although in my personal opinion, there is never enough wine). Lack of desire is often a hormone issue that needs to be treated, monitored, and adjusted by your urologist. Rarely, it can be an anatomical issue that requires an expert like the doctor, who can examine the patient and remedy the problem. Add into the mix that each woman is very unique in her sexual desires and then throw in the fact that it always seems to boil down to how she "feels". A woman's mood is a complicated subject and central to her sexuality. Most women understand this about themselves but may struggle to communicate it to their partner. Simply giving yourself permission to explore this other dimension of your own sexuality will help you to understand your own way to achieve great sex and deep satisfaction.

Now, being the plumber's wife, I always have questions about why I cannot just go to my gynecologist to have my hormones adjusted, or better yet, fixed. At this point, the plumber must be called a "plumber" for the simple fact that women do not identify with owning a penis. However, all women identify with plumbing issues and that has everything to do with urine and sex.

We understand when there is an issue with the plumbing down there and we realize that anything could be wrong. It's so complex that it is hard to know where to start. The plumber doctor informs me of several reasons why I must go to a urologist like him. A popular reason is that a urologist is specifically trained to treat patients with lack of desire as it can potentially have several root causes. Anything from anatomy to psychology to hormones. Who knew?!

Because a lack of desire is a type of sexual dysfunction, a urologist is specifically trained in sexual dysfunction. Yes, this is a certifiable problem and doctors are specifically trained in sexual medicine. Heck, I get a magazine in the mail every month titled "Society of Sexual Medicine." My mailman always hand delivers my mail with a very large grin on his face on the day this magazine arrives. I cannot tell if he is just being nice or if he is secretly wishing to meet the doctor for a personal consultation. I must admit that I do chuckle when the mailman rings the bell to hand me the monthly magazine.

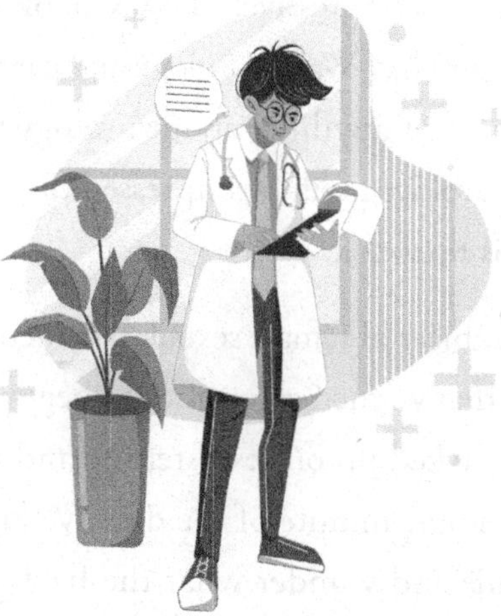

A urologist is very different from the obstetrician/gynecologist, who is trained to help you grow your babies and deliver them. The gynecologist is also the doctor that helps you to believe that you can get through the entire process successfully. A urologist is specifically trained in sexual medicine and all the moving parts that make it happen, which are many more parts than what the gynecologist is trained to know about. If you would like more information on all the urological parts versus gynecological parts, there is a medical textbook called "Campbell's Urology." This is the book that taught the doctor everything he initially learned about urology. My girlfriend Barbara was one of the illustrators for this textbook, which makes my world very small and somewhat entertaining. You will also be entertained once you see all her drawings. Kudos to you, Barbara. Impressive! The textbook has since been renamed Campbell-Walsh Urology and can be found online. It will answer anything about urology and your board-certified urologist will be impressed that you even know about this textbook.

The unspoken subject of female sexual dysfunction is not really a subject that women care about to begin with. It's not like we are jacked up on testosterone and ready for action at every single minute of the day. We know men who are like this and wonder what the heck is wrong with them and accuse them of having a one-track mind.

Sexual dysfunction among the female population is usually missed completely. A woman often just believes that she is over exhausted from taking care of everyone and everything, or she simply believes that she is no longer in love or lust with her man. In some rare instances, a woman may not be in love with her partner anymore due to issues like addiction, obesity, chasing other women, or being gone all the time. With those exceptions aside, sexual dysfunction is a condition that is often missed, or worse yet, never properly identified and treated. Female sexual dysfunction has a very specific set of criteria that makes it a bit easier to identify. Once you identify if you are suffering from sexual dysfunction, you now know that it can be treated!

The reason this subject is more important than just sex is because a healthy sexual lifestyle is a very important part of a solid relationship and plays a big role in your overall health and happiness. There is plenty of research out there that shows the benefits of a healthy sexual lifestyle. Sex brings balance to life and is as natural as the birds and the bees. It is also something special to be experienced and enjoyed. This element of life does make a difference in your overall wellness, hence the study of sexual medicine. Sex is medicine.

I had a very dear girlfriend who married a truly great guy. He was head over heels for her and she with him. They ended up having two babies in just three years. About a year after having the second baby, the relationship started to become incredibly strained. One would think it was just the stress of two small children. However, it was more than that. Lack of desire had taken over my girlfriend.

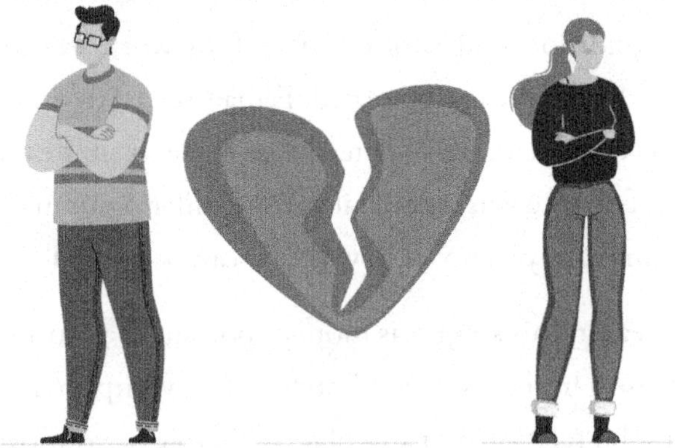

Initially, she thought that she was just exhausted from motherhood and work. That is an incredibly exhausting schedule. Add to it a husband and a missing sex life, combined with not enough money in the bank, and you would think that was a temporary problem. However, it turned out that her hormones were out of whack without her knowledge. She was convinced that she was tired and simply not interested in sex. This was not such a big deal to her, but it was a very big deal to her husband. Over time, the issue overtook the marriage and arguments began to increase along with the responsibility of work and children.

There wasn't any more sex in the marriage to clear the mind and relax the body and keep the marriage vital. Both parties were simply unhappy and not really understanding that the wife's lack of desire was a medical problem and not just an exhaustion issue. Lack of desire won this battle, and I am sad to report that they eventually divorced when the kids were just three and four years old. This divorce was most likely the result of undiagnosed sexual dysfunction. The gynecologist missed it, the wife missed it, and the husband missed it.

My girlfriend never knew about a urologist, let alone about sexual dysfunction. She was too tired and too disinterested to even consider that there was help available to get her sex life back and create the balancing act of marriage and family. Years later, she did address her hormone problem at the young age of 40 and realized that perhaps the root cause of her divorce was actually a medical problem.

Let's look at some of the items on the checklist of sexual dysfunction and see if you are suffering from any of the them.

The first and most obvious to identify is sex that hurts like hell, no matter which angle you put it in. It seems the harder you try to find just the right angle; you are sure to make it hurt even more. The good news here is that you are not crazy. Sex is truly not working anymore because of possibly both physical and physiological changes to your body over time. With this condition, many women get to the point where they decide that sex is just not necessary and certainly not worth it anymore. And this is where the relationship problems begin to boil under the surface. The high level of discomfort, combined with the physical and emotional demands from your partner, create a level of stress that could probably rival any nuclear reactor on the planet.

The second item on the list is low arousal. This is most likely not news to you and is the absolute lack of interest in anything sexual. You've probably even said if you never had sex again that would be too soon. You're laughing out loud right now because you either said it or your girlfriends have. This subject of low arousal probably does not sound out of the ordinary to you, nor did you probably realize that it is a part of sexual dysfunction. Heck, getting laid once a month is more than plenty, right? You'll be relieved to know that most women have experienced low arousal at some point in their lives.

If you want confirmation that you may be suffering from low arousal, simply try a variety of items to try and get yourself aroused. There are a host of sexual cues to choose from and everybody likes something different. You could get right to the point and watch pornography with your significant other in the privacy of your own love nest. Or you can have some fun with a little experiment to see if you can get a little turned on or excited and generate some exciting sexual thoughts. If you would like to test this out without your significant other, try the hot fireman's calendar or watch the half-naked man walking around the set of every soap opera on TV. Maybe you like soldiers in action like me, or perhaps you are more of a voyeur and like to relax at a fancy hotel swimming pool in Las Vegas where the odds are in your favor to see something delicious walk by that is sure to make you wet. No, I am not talking about peeing your pants, yet.

By now, you probably have a visual of what you like to see and perhaps remember what it was like to feel aroused by the images you were able to recall. That is arousal. That is the magic that occurs in your brain so the rest of the body parts will follow. Science has shown us that 99% of an orgasm starts in the brain and it ends in the best place on earth, deep inside your body that is almost impossible to explain where and when it happens. It is just awesome, and the best part is that when you are done, an orgasm is equivalent to a great workout and a top-notch facial. With all that blood pulsing through your body, it's no wonder you look and feel 10 years younger. There is no health drink on the planet that can rival the miraculous orgasm.

The final problem with sexual dysfunction is the inability to achieve an orgasm. Do you remember what those are ladies? Just refer to the last paragraph and relive the glory and reignite those desires deep inside you. If you are still feeling nothing stirring around inside of you, this is a good indication to get to a urologist who specializes in sexual dysfunction so you can enjoy an orgasm again. They are an important part of having a healthy sexual life and are one of the greatest gifts here on earth. They take you away to a place of complete satisfaction without a care in the world. They leave you clear-headed, happy, content, and ready to take on the world.

Another reason to go see a urologist is to rule out any potential health issues that may be the root cause for your specific sexual dysfunction. There are several physical issues that can get in the way of a healthy sex life. The most prevalent one is hormonal imbalance. Most women realize there is a hormone level change that occurs mainly after menopause. Your problem could be that simple. Those hormones you complained about during your baby making years had a much bigger role than just growing babies. They were the secret sauce to achieving sexual desire and orgasm.

When a woman's estrogen level drops for any particular health reason, this dramatically reduces the amount of good blood flow to the female body parts down below where all the magic happens. If you don't have good blood flow down there, the tissue ends up being less receptive and ready for action. You may also have another problem down there with low estrogen levels. The magic cave starts to dry out making anything sliding along those fantastic walls of the vagina seem like torture. Estrogen is the magic hormone that keeps the vaginal tissue plump and wet. Anything less is just unpleasant and can make having sex feel more painful and unpleasant.

There are some women who may also suffer from what is called Hypoactive Sexual Desire Disorder. It's less common and a bit harder to diagnose. This is when women have problems in their sex life that cannot be explained. A good urologist will provide what is called standard of care and follow all the protocols to try and diagnose your sexual dysfunction. However, after trying pills, creams, and thorough examinations to rule out other health issues, the woman may still suffer from sexual dysfunction. This is an extreme situation, but it does occur.

Sexual dysfunction for women is more common than for men. What's the problem? Hormones usually. There are different categories of sexual dysfunction like pelvic pain, and the number one is lack of desire, which can be both hormonal or the way a woman "feels" about sex. Why go to a urologist instead of a gynecologist? Because gynecologists are not trained to treat sexual dysfunction. So, ladies, go find a board-certified urologist to help you address these issues.

So, what do you do for lack of desire? Take your hormones to keep your desire and body functioning, a.k.a., staying wet! You may not realize that there is a problem and it's not an easy discussion to have with your lover. Women are pleasers and try to fix things on their own. Toss out this unnecessary burden and get to your urologist. Don't forget to ponder your own feelings about sex and enjoy the complexity of your female nature and use it to your advantage in the bedroom with your new hormone prescription.

Discover your own stars.

Chapter 20

SKIN CREAM COMPANIES – MOISTURIZE THIS!

Wave that magic wand down there

The global skin care market is a multi-billion-dollar business and that is because society believes that a few wrinkles on our face, neck or hands will somehow negatively affect a person's perception of our appearance. It is believed that if you purchase the "best" skin care line, all your aging beauty problems will be solved, and your youth shall somehow be preserved. The truth is that your youth is not just the smooth plump skin on your face, neck, or hands, but your youth is also your plumbing down there. It turns out that your vagina needs as much moisturizing and attention as your face, neck, and hands after menopause. Yes, we all hate the "V" word. But it deserves as much attention as your face.

In 2013, which seems like yesterday, the International Society for the Study of Women's Sexual Health (ISSWSH), and the North American Menopause Society (NAMS), got together and decided to update the way we label a woman's vaginal plumbing issues. The old terms like atrophic vaginitis and vulvovaginal atrophy were tossed out. The reason for this was because we have learned that there are more parts to your plumbing that need to be a part of the same conversation in order for you to keep your quality of life when you hit menopause.

The new term that is used is call Genitourinary Syndrome of Menopause (GSM). If your doctor is not familiar with this term, then get another doctor because that means they are not reading all the current research being done to improve a woman's plumbing in an effort to preserve her quality of life during menopause. Research has proven that low dose estrogen in many forms is beneficial for solving GSM symptoms.

Hormone Replacement Therapy is no longer a bad word. We know so much more today. With proper monitoring and a physician who is current with his or her training and certifications, understands that hormone replacement benefits far outweigh the risks. Risks are now mitigated because we know how to properly monitor a patient using hormone replacement therapy. Whether you are using systemic estrogen, which is administered several ways such as a pill, injection, patch, pellet, or applying cream to your skin, or you are using local estrogen in the vagina, it can be done safely under a doctor's care. Patients simply need to keep their scheduled appointments and follow their physician's instructions. Your physician will work with you to provide the safest form of estrogen for your personal battle with GSM.

The prevalence of GSM is under recognized, undertreated, and under discussed between a woman and her physician. Most women believe that the symptoms of GSM are a natural part of aging and menopause. That is just wrong! Physicians are the front-line providers and must reevaluate the way they view a woman's quality of life issues when faced with GSM symptoms. It seems that doctors are just not good at asking these kinds of screening questions because it has always been accepted that hormone replacement therapy is bad and that leaking urine and having vaginal discomfort is a normal aging process. This is just not true and the research backs this up.

By shining a light on GSM and adding one of the many GSM treatments to your daily beauty regiment of skin care using a variety of creams, quality of life can be returned by adding one more cream for down there.

The subject of GSM brings us right back to your skin care routine. If you think soap, water, and face cream are important, wait until you learn the benefits of putting on your cream down there. Imagine making the upper half of your body gorgeous, while the lower half is dry, irritated, itchy, leaky, stinky, and always left with a sense of frequency and urgency. Your lower half can now be as functional and beautiful as your upper half. Women who do not seek the simple and affordable treatments available today are highly unlikely to achieve sexual satisfaction and retain a quality of life. Add to this the fact that you will also be faced with urinary changes in the lower genital tract, which is code for repetitive urinary tract infections, and you have a recipe for being unhappy and chasing down the next toilet every day of your life.

So, what happens when GSM sets in with menopause. First of all, the symptoms that start to present are in no way life threatening. However, they do have a direct impact on your day to day quality of life and have been described by affected women as a chronic condition down there that alters their quality of life. The estrogen that circulates throughout the body during a woman's younger days and before menopause is what keeps the vaginal walls and urinary track plump and lubricated and ready to respond to the need to pee or that awesome pleasing sensation during sex.

Because estrogen plays a large role in urinary continence it is important that you are always able to empty your bladder each time you pee, or you can develop a urinary tract infection. Without proper levels of estrogen, this becomes an Olympic feat. Also, when estrogen is low or missing it becomes almost impossible to control your urethra and stop peeing on command. At some point during menopause, you will leak urine without even knowing it until you check your panties or start to smell yourself.

Your connective tissues down there need estrogen the same way a bodybuilder needs food to function. The same is true for the tissues and organs involved in your sexual function. When estrogen is no longer present, sexual dysfunction shows up in the form of a decrease in collagen and tissue elasticity, along with fewer blood vessels. This change in lowered or missing estrogen starts GSM symptoms such as vaginal dryness, irritation (both vaginal and attitude), itching, tenderness, bleeding during sex and pain when the big erection shows up to the party. Estrogen is a key ingredient to a woman's fight against the negative impact of Genitourinary Syndrome of Menopause (GSM).

It turns out that estrogen and estrogen receptors have a very big job to do in a woman's body. It seems that we still know very little about how the molecular mechanisms of estrogen actually work and where they impact a woman's body. So far, science seems to believe that estrogen and estrogen receptors have many jobs in the body such as keeping healthy skin, hair, bones, tissue, muscles and all things cardiovascular. Most research has been done on the link between estrogen and cancer. This seems to be where the “big scare” about hormone replacement therapy got its legs. We are now swinging the pendulum the other direction and discovering that low doses of estrogen in menopause are very beneficial but simply require regular monitoring by your physician.

Knowing that estrogen and estrogen receptors play an important role in both your urological and gynecological health during menopause opens the door to getting your quality of life back by being open to the many solutions available for low dose hormone treatment.

The key understanding for me when trying to understand what the heck was happening during menopause became very clear when I learned this one thing. Evidently there are estrogen receptors throughout your body including your human plumbing. These estrogen receptors are simply waiting for estrogen present in the woman’s body to tell the receptors what to do. These receptors are in the bladder and urethra as well as your gynecological plumbing, which is in charge of sexual function. The estrogen circulates through your system and essentially tells the receptors “what to flex or activate”. This messaging system between estrogen and estrogen receptors is what activates your reflex to pee or not to pee. When there is a deficiency with estrogen in your system, there is no way to tell the estrogen receptors to do their job. Therefore, both your urological and gynecological health start to dwindle and all the working tissues and muscles slow down and seize to function properly.

We still do not know enough about the benefits of the molecular mechanism of estrogen and the estrogen receptors. We do know that these estrogen receptors are present in the bladder and urethra, as well as the sexual function real estate. It is necessary to have a level of estrogen present in a woman's body telling the receptors what to do and minimize the effects of GSM. The only way to achieve this goal for women is to raise the awareness among women and their physicians so they both understand the benefits of locally applied estrogen and how it can change the game in the fight against GSM.

Now that you have a clear understanding of GSM and low estrogen therapies to improve your quality of life without risking your health, let me share the estrogen stories of both myself and my twin sister. As I was writing this book, I would share my book with my twin sister, as she was always interested in my project and would never lie to me about how good or bad it was. For those of you who know Helen, you are probably laughing and nodding your head right now.

Helen and I were on speaker phone one evening discussing our personal hormone replacement therapies, while the Doctor who was standing nearby, listened in to our phone call. We were discussing this chapter and the effects of estrogen. Both Helen and I take our estrogen differently. She uses local low dose estrogen and I use a topical combination of creams and a pill, which would be considered systemic estrogen therapy.

Helen asked me where I put my cream and how much I use. I told her that I rub the cream on my shoulder like the doctor does when he applies his testosterone. I love the effects of his testosterone, but that's another chapter! I put the estrogen on my shoulder because there were no instructions on the label to direct me how to use it. The Doctor jumped right into the conversation and demanded to know if my gynecologist had instructed me on how to use it. I thought this was a silly question, since he was obviously agitated at my level of ignorance about where to put the cream and already knew I was doing it wrong. With his tense voice demanding a correct answer, I was smart enough to ask, "where should I be putting it?"

The Doctor immediately demonstrated exactly where I should have been rubbing the cream in to. He jams his left hand up inside his inner thigh and probably scared it out of his left testicle during the demonstration. I was shocked to learn that the cream goes on my inner thigh. Evidently, the inner thigh area is a better absorption point for women. I should have guessed that since that is a wonderfully sensitive location on Friday night date night!

It turns out that I have been rubbing this damn cream on my shoulder for almost a year already. I was an excellent patient and made it to each of my checkups for my bloodwork and interview about how the hormones were working. My dosage had been changed twice as my numbers were a bit low. Now I know why my estrogen numbers were low. I was applying the damn cream to my shoulder, which is a low absorption area for women. It is these small details that make women feel like second class citizens. You would think as the Doctor's wife, that I would have either known better or been caught in the act of doing it wrong much sooner.

With regards to the missing instructions on my prescription bottle and the detailed instructions or demonstration from my doctor on how to use the product correctly, that was a problem. It would have been fantastic to be fully educated on my war against GSM. I am sure that my doctor assumed that the Doctor would have already told me how to use the stuff. Clearly, that never happened and I of all people, was as ignorant as most other women who suffer from GSM like me.

My twin sister proceeds to tell me that she also had no instructions on her prescription tube. She had no idea how to exactly place her estrogen in a very strategic location. She also did not have instructions on how much to use or when. Evidently, it is best to apply the cream at night before bed. Helen was a bit worried about using estrogen at all so on her own volition, she decided to just use it twice a week without really understanding the consequences of self-prescribing. When the Doctor heard this information, he was again agitated at the lack of education between physician and patient, when it comes to getting hormone replacement therapy right.

In order to achieve optimal results from low dose vaginal estrogen, it must be applied every other day. The amount should be specified by your doctor and placed on the prescription label. If the doctor tells you to use it three times a week, then please use it three times a week. This is an important part of the treatment plan. It would have helped my sister had the doctor taken the time during her appointment to clearly explain why three times a week is necessary and demonstrate exactly where to put the cream, how much cream and how deep it must be inserted. You try messing around down there with a cream and no instructions and then walk around with it all day long. These are the small things that can either make your life easy or hard. This is a great example as to how education shall set you free. Where have we heard that before? Thank you, Oprah!

The other question that my twin sister asked was if the estrogen cream that she was using would cause any side effects for her husband? What a great question. I had an instant visual of his penis shrinking, and instantly growing man boobs on their date nights. Luckily, the Doctor informed us both that there were no side effects for the partner when coming in contact with any of the estrogen creams that a woman may apply to her body, whether it is the inner thigh, vagina or the shoulder.

These issues are just several of the problems with getting doctors up to date about treating GSM. More conversations need to be had about educating women and physicians on GSM and going through the steps together with the patient to educate and prescribe the correct forms of estrogen customized for each patient. These treatments work and are needed to reduce symptoms of GSM that may impact your quality of life.

GSM is a chronic disorder that will not improve without some intervention and treatment. Women have come to accept this as aging. This is more LIES. I am encouraging you to consider having this discussion with a knowledgeable doctor who is educated about all facets of GSM and find a way to help you. Don't hesitate to act. You owe it to yourself to inquire, educate, act, and feel better.

I hope I have the attention of women, pharmaceutical companies, and skin care manufacturers. We should all unite in an effort to educate, research and treat GSM, making treatments available to women around the world, the same way that skin care companies have infiltrated every single woman's psyche about her face, neck, and hands.

Remember that half of the planet is female, and half of those women probably already have some form of cream from a major skin care company. GSM should be discussed ad nauseum. It is normal and OK to discuss how to safely moisturize and treat the menopausal vagina with low dose hormones.

According to the 2010 United States census, there are approximately 50 million women in the U.S. Alone who are over the age of 51[2,3], which is the average age of menopause. That is a lot of cream, whether it's for your hands or your vagina! Sadly, one study found that very few physicians inquired about GSM Symptoms in their female patients. The hesitation to prescribe treatment combined with patient concerns over safety of topical vaginal therapies, keep this subject under wraps. That is just crazy when GSM can be clinically detected in up to 90% of postmenopausal women[4]. Women go above and beyond there already busy lives to go to the doctor

2 Howden LM, Julia. Age and Sex Composition: 2010. In. Commerce USDo, trans. United States Census Bureau: U.S. Census Bureau; 2010.

3 Avis NE, McKinlay SM. The Massachusetts Women's Health Study: an epidemiologic investigation of the menopause. J Am Med Womens Assoc (1972). 1995;50(2):45-49, 63

4 Palacios S, Nappi RE, Bruyniks N, Particco M, Panay N, Investigators ES. The European Vulvovaginal Epidemiological Survey (EVES): prevalence, symptoms and impact of vulvovaginal atrophy of menopause. Climacteric. 2018;21(3):286-291.

for checkups. It's time to start this conversation and get updated on the current research being done on low dose estrogen therapies to treat GSM.

Low estrogen issues are often not recognized by most women as a reason for their lower urinary tract issues or vaginal discomfort. Genital Symptoms, Sexual Symptoms, and Urinary Symptoms can be treated similarly the same way you treat your face, neck and hands with creams. The only difference is that the cream for down there has a little extra kick to it for your quality of life issues with regards to your plumbing and vaginal comfort.

With regular visits to your urologist or gynecologist, treating GSM is no different than a mammogram or cholesterol checkup. An appropriate effective therapy for GSM should be a part of every menopausal woman's care and beauty regimen. The only difference when adding a low dose estrogen cream is scheduling regular visits to your board-certified urologist or gynecologist, who is familiar with Genitourinary Syndrome of Menopause (GSM).

I can remember when my twin sister and I were much younger, and our grandparents would come to visit. My grandma would spend lots of time getting ready and we would stand at her side in the bathroom as she went through her beauty routine. The one thing that I remembered, and it always made me laugh was the final touch of perfume at the end. She would squirt some perfume on her neck, a little on her wrists, and a last spritz between the legs for good measure! I always wondered why she did that.

As I got older, I learned that due to the above-mentioned symptoms of GSM, a woman's crotch could be subjected to unpleasant odors due to leaking urine or undetected urinary tract infections. We are beyond the days of spritzing our crotch with perfume. Be brave and start the conversation with your doctor. If your doctor is unaware of GSM, give them a copy of this book and go find yourself an up to date physician who truly cares about your urological and menopausal health.

One study found that just 13% of physicians inquired about GSM symptoms amongst their patients[5]. Even after the patient was found to have symptoms, most women would continue to go untreated, despite the effects on their quality of life issues. The resistance to prescribing low dose estrogen is an outdated approach and is a red flag to alert you as to whether your physician has stayed current with the most recent research and benefits of low dose estrogen. Estrogen is not a bad word. It is the key ingredient for a woman to regain her quality of life with regards to her urological plumbing issues and sexual health.

---

5 Portman DJ, Gass ML. Genitourinary syndrome of menopause: new terminology for vulvovaginal atrophy from the International Society for the Study of Women's Sexual Health and the North American Menopause Society. Maturitas. 2014;79(3):349-354.

Although many women believe that hormonal therapies come with inherent risks, this is no longer the case for most women using low dose estrogen in some form. Make the time to go have a discussion with your board-certified urologist or gynecologist, who is current with the latest research and proper applications of low dose estrogen. Do not listen to TV commercials trying to sell you anything to do with your hormones. Leave this to a physician only. Just imagine improving your quality of life by adding one simple step to your beauty routine. Although many women are not happy with the inconvenience of inserting one more thing in there, the benefits far outweigh the complaining.

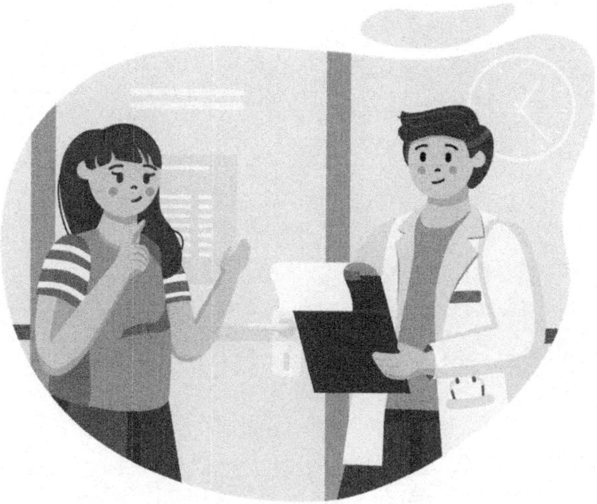

For all of you men who made it through this chapter, if your wife is not calling her doctor, go ahead and start dialing. One more cream in the house will be an amazing addition to your relationship. Face, Neck, and hand creams are great when the lights are on, but cream for down there is awesome when the lights are off. You will benefit greatly by being by her side and supporting her through the gauntlet of information that she will be overwhelmed by. Estrogen therapy not only improves the quality of life for a woman but improves the quality of the relationship for the man. Estrogen is your friend, and remember, rub it on the inner thigh, not the shoulder!

Chapter 21

SEX TIPS FOR YOUR NEW PLUMBING

The unknown lights up the soul when fear is conquered

Now because we just covered the chapter on lack of desire and you found out that the doctor is a sexual medicine expert, you may have more questions to explore with regards to sex. My first advice is to make sure that your board-certified urologist has got you in good working order, that all of your sexual plumbing is ready for action, and your hormone levels are appropriate for your health situation. After that, it is up to you and your partner to explore your physical delights in a mutually agreeable way and carve out a new path to physical pleasures that excite you both. The Doctor is not a sex doctor, but a plumber who is skilled at getting your sex organs in good working order. Once you are plumbed properly and no leaks are occurring and the lube levels are satisfactory, you are set to rock each other's world.

I bring this section up in the book because my twin sister felt as though there needed to be an entire chapter on sex tips. I thought this to be an odd request as I know that a urologist is not a sex coach. Evidently, my sister thinks the doctor is close to sainthood on this subject. It must be due to all of the conversations we've had over the years about all things marriage.

My sister helped me to clearly delineate the role of a urologist and what it has to do exactly with your sex life. A urologist can address the physical issues with your sex organs and most likely repair those organs or get them back to proper function. However, a good urologist does not give out sex tips for achieving orgasms. That is up to you and your partner as you explore the bandwidth of your updated urological plumbing. This is your chance to discover your own stars.

Chapter 22

GO SEE A UROLOGIST OR UROGYNECOLOGIST

Now you know the top three most prevalent urological problems for men and women. This is just the tip of the iceberg with regards to all things urology. We now know that the top 3 issues for men are lack of desire, erectile dysfunction and prostate problems. The top 3 issues for women are incontinence, pelvic prolapse, and lack of desire. Any of these conditions should only be treated by a board-certified urologist who is current in their training and understanding of the newest and most effective ways to take care of your urological health. There is a solution for all urological problems that each of us may face at some point during our lifetimes.

My message to all men and women would be "GO SEE A UROLOGIST OR UROGYNECOLOGIST." The Doctor tells me that patients wait too long to seek help.

Women are used to dealing with discomfort and often don't make the time to care for themselves properly until it becomes a crisis, like peeing during an orgasm. Men seem to wait until they are already peeing blood. The faster you get to your board-certified urologist or urogynecologist, the better. Your quality of life is waiting for you to grab the phone and call your board-certified urologist or urogynecologist.

Chapter 23

PELVIC THERAPY – NO NOT THAT KIND

Learning is a gift like no other

As curiosity would have it, I had to ask a really good question of the Doctor. I wanted to know how he could tell when a woman needed to have pelvic physical therapy versus surgery. My question was not actually a good one as this is not an either-or situation. The complexity of determining whether a woman can get away with simple physical therapy versus a potential surgery can only be determined by a thorough examination by your urologist. Of course, I had to ask what the initial clue was that would alert the doctor to know what to do. This question led to a conversation that took me into a virtual exam room that I wished I had never entered.

I have never really taken the time to stop and think about what the doctor actually does day in and day out. Honestly, I simply have a visual of him in the operating room with that silly hair net and scrubs covered in spatters of blood. That visual alone is enough to make any further thoughts simply cease. You can imagine my shock and surprise when the doctor started to tell me about what he must do in order to determine next steps for either pelvic physical therapy or a potential surgery. The Doctors nonchalantly starts to tell me that he must examine a female patient by sticking his fingers in her vagina and asking her to "squeeze" his fingers. I am pretty damn sure that I did not hear another word after that, as I was utterly shocked that the doctor was testing out vaginas all day long. I knew he was fixing penises, I just never realized he was an expert with vaginas too.

Moving on, the Doctor continues to tell me that when a woman cannot squeeze his fingers during the exam, he will often schedule them to be seen by his pelvic floor physical therapist for pelvic floor therapy, which can include exercises such as Kegel exercises. These are the most well-known, all the way to pelvic floor physical therapy. At this point, I made the Doctor back up and restate what he had just said. I then proceeded to ask why he would ask them to squeeze his fingers. The Doctor tells me that the majority of the time a woman does not squeeze his fingers, but instead squeezes her buttocks or belly in an effort to squeeze his fingers, which renders the verdict of a nonexistent pelvic muscle, hence incontinence, or even pelvic prolapse.

As soon as I found out that the doctor had a pelvic floor physical therapist, I immediately needed to meet this individual and conduct an interview to learn everything there was to know about the world of pelvic floor physical therapy. I asked the doctor to hook me up with his physical therapist as soon as possible so I could extract every piece of information available to solve pelvic floor failure and incontinence in both women and men. I approached this gentleman as though he was the up and coming star on the red carpet.

I met Dr. Alex on a busy morning at the office. I wanted to see if he actually had a following of patients who needed his services. Dr. Alex was right on time and very happy to welcome me into his therapy room where all the magic happened for patients suffering from leaking pipes. As we entered the exam room, Dr. Alex was very welcoming and also delighted that I would be interested in what he was doing to add to our practice. I made it clear to Dr. Alex, how thrilled I was to know that he had joined our practice and was adding one more valuable resource for the doctor's patients. I then had to remind Dr. Alex that I was simply the wife and not a doctor so please go slowly and be patient with my questions, as they may be a bit ignorant.

At first glance, the exam room seemed to be like any other medical exam room, with the exception of a few items.

There was some simple exercise equipment like medicine balls, stretch bands and very light weights. Little did I know that the most intimidating piece of equipment in the room would end up being the computer. I should have noted the wires with electrodes on the end shooting out from the computer. These are eventually placed in very strategic locations to train the brain on how to get the muscles down there to respond correctly and repeatedly in an effort to train them and strengthen them.

Dr. Alex proceeded to tell me that urology is the busiest practice in our town which confirmed that just about everyone has some type of urological problem, both men and women, and reaffirmed why I rarely see the doctor. Pelvic floor therapy is not gender specific and is applied to men and women equally.

I focused on Dr. Alex like a chemist in a lab trying to discover the secret to science. After all, we were both on a mission. I needed to write this book and he needed to educate people about his services and how he could help them. I was wonderfully surprised at how Dr. Alex lit up like a Christmas tree just like the doctor with the thought that I had a urological question for him.

I started our appointment by bringing up the last conversation I had with my childhood girlfriend and the efficacy of her medical experiment with Ben Wa Balls. But just like the doctor, Dr. Alex did not know what Ben Wa Balls were either. He thought they were French. I am not sure where that came from, but it made me laugh. Without hesitation, I jumped right in and started to educate him on this newfound tool for his trade. He likened them to internal weights. I liked his description very much and will most likely use this description for any future conversations with my girlfriend.

Dr. Alex proceeded to breeze by my Ben Wa Balls inquiry and got back to the real business of pelvic floor physical therapy and all it has to offer for both men and women. He began to show off the tools of the trade. He explained the purpose of the exam table was so the patient could start the basic pelvic floor exercises while lying down, which was to remove the effects of gravity pulling on any of the pelvic floor muscles. This position allows the patient to properly identify the pelvic muscles and then proceed to the task of strengthening the pelvic floor.

After graduating from the horizontal position on the exam table, the patient can then progress to the sitting position while doing the recommended physical therapy exercises. Once the sitting position is mastered and strengthened, and muscles lengthened and relaxed, the patient can then graduate to the standing position while doing therapy. The standing position allows the patient to continue to strengthen the pelvic floor muscles, so it becomes possible again to do floor exercises while standing, squatting, lunging, and even running and jumping. These basic exercises cause heavy leakage in patients with incontinence issues and reduces quality of life. Pelvic floor physical therapy is a winner winner chicken dinner for anyone who leaks.

The main thing Dr. Alex stressed was the ability to learn how to relax and strengthen the pelvic floor muscles so they can function properly. He uses gravity as one of his tools for strength training. He focuses on lengthening the muscles, getting stronger, and eventually achieving a better resting and toned muscle status for the pelvic floor. In the end, the patient has a naturally relaxed pelvic floor muscle because it is now stronger and can hold up the uterus and bladder the way it did when the patient was much younger.

This newly achieved status allows patients to go out into the world and shake their booty without leaking or possibly having their organs slide right out onto the dance floor. Achieving continence should be the new status that every person would want to achieve and shout out to the world, "look at me, I don't leak pee!"

Remember the computer in the exam room? Well this is the little gem with electrodes shooting out from it which strategically connects to very specific locations that can detect muscle movement and muscle strength in the pelvic floor. Biofeedback is a very effective way for the patient to see the progress they are making with the exercises assigned for pelvic floor physical therapy. Although this approach seems a bit intimidating, Dr. Alex shared that it is his patients' favorite part of therapy because they can now see the progress they are making toward continence.

Posture! We can all hear our mother telling us to stand up straight at some point in our life. Now that you are older and probably leaking, you know that your mother was right. Dr. Alex said that when a person has bad posture or an inward curve in their lower back while standing, this can slightly squeeze the bladder and aggravate the nerves in the lower back. Just picture a person standing with their butt cheeks sticking outward. This position causes pressure on your insides and can aggravate the nerves that control the bladder. Aggravated bladder nerves are the winning ticket for incontinence in some cases. Who knew there was a correct posture to help with bladder control?

The correct posture to promote healthy bladder control is to have a little bit of a forward posterior pelvic tilt, while shoulders remain straight. Think of it as though you are sticking your penis slightly out and forward. Ladies, for this exercise, you will have to strap one on in your mind. You can do it. Now imagine just slightly showing off that penis and sticking it a little bit forward, while keeping your back and shoulders straight. That is the magic position for good posture with regards to your plumbing. This slight adjustment in your posture can make a difference over time and strengthen your core muscles needed to keep that pelvic floor strong.

Now this is the part you have all been waiting for! What actually happens during the physical therapy consultation for your urological crisis? It starts off like most other physical therapy consultations. The physical therapist has you lie on the exam table and checks to see how your joints are able to move. This is because the physical therapist wants to make sure you can use your gluteal muscles (butt cheeks) and that you can move your knees and hips. These muscles are involved in strengthening the pelvic floor. After movability and strength are determined, the physical therapist may use a medicine ball as a tool to check and see if you are able rest your lower legs up on top of the ball while lying down. He or she will then ask you to try and move your hips and knees. At the same time, the physical therapist may ask you to try and squeeze your Kegel muscles while moving your legs. This kind of conditioning may sound simple, but if you are a leaker, you are already worried about the puddle that is beginning to form underneath you.

The second phase of the physical therapy becomes a bit more intimate after your basic strength assessment and movability tests are complete. The doctor will ask you to

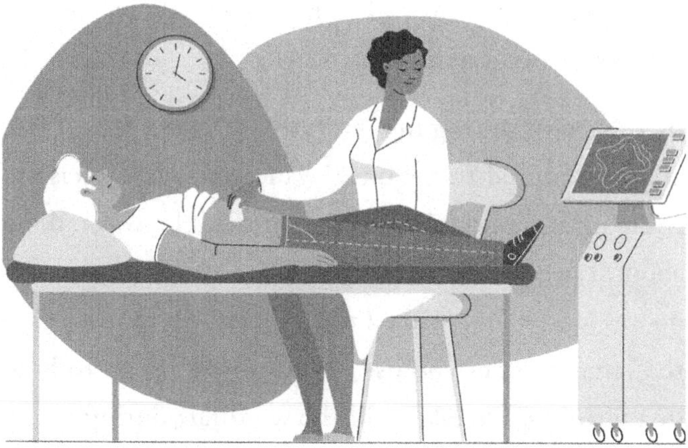

remove your pants and will use a form of biofeedback that will now move you toward a mind body connection. By hooking up sensors from a computer monitor to your external genitals initially, the physical therapist will guide you on finding the proper muscles to contract and release in an effort to mentally find your pelvic floor muscles and then engage them properly. The purpose for the initial external setup is to minimize your discomfort. The doctor is still able to achieve results working in this manner. Eventually, you will progress and so will those electrodes.

As you are doing biofeedback, there is a computer monitor that displays the muscle response values as you contract and release the pelvic floor muscles. The physical therapist will explain to not move the back or hips and focus on trying to contract and release the pelvic floor. The computer monitor will reinforce what is correct and will not respond when it is incorrect.

At this point during my interview with Dr. Alex, I was almost tempted to try out the biofeedback exercise to really understand which damn muscles he was talking about. I needed more clarity as to exactly which muscles he was after. He informed me that the exact muscles are the same muscles you use when you are trying to hold in a fart. Yes, Dr. Alex said the word fart during a very serious interview. However, Dr. Alex said this word with such soft precision that he actually made the word "fart" sound as though it were the harp in an orchestra.

As soon as Dr. Alex described how to find the pelvic floor muscle by describing the intense resistance to not fart, a light bulb went off in my head and I immediately understood exactly where the pelvic floor muscle was located. If I were the doctor, I would tell you to go home and eat the foods that make you fart like a rock star so you can practice holding in your farts as part of your pelvic floor rehabilitation. Everything became so simple so fast with the thought of having to hold in my farts.

I now realized that every time I went to the nursing home to visit my mom and was hearing farts flying around the place like a New York traffic jam, it all had to do with pelvic floor muscles. It was always amazing how the residents would simply be walking down the hallways, farting with every step, all the way to the dining room. The interesting part was that they either didn't hear the fart, feel the fart, or simply care that they were farting at all. Well, now I know they were suffering from weak pelvic floor muscles that couldn't hold in a fart, let alone urine. The secret fix to improving continence has now been revealed to me and gave me an idea for a bumper sticker, "Resist the fart and stop the leak."

During the biofeedback therapy, the physical therapist continues to instruct the patient to squeeze the pelvic floor muscles as though they were holding in that walking fart. With this thought in mind and the intention to do so, the patient can see the computer monitor respond with a flicker of movement for contracting and releasing the right muscles. At that very moment, the patient can make a mind body connection and feel like they got it right. Dr. Alex will ask them to look at the movement on the monitor and at the same time try to remember what it felt like squeezing that muscle and immediately repeat it correctly. The mind body connection is made and then the work begins to strengthen the desired muscle. That type of both physical and mental confirmation helps to train the pelvic floor muscles.

The one thing to remember about pelvic floor physical therapy is that it focuses on the entire person, which includes good posture, joint care for your knees, and finding your Kegel muscles. The final stage of urological physical therapy is the computer feedback for making that mind and muscle connection as you continue to strengthen the correct muscles. You will progress to marching in place and eventually get stronger, better, and drier. Patients who follow the doctor's orders will see results.

There is good news with this type of a workout, because like with any other workout routine, you are able to see some results in about 6 to 8 weeks. However, if the patient continues to hold in farts, follow the exercises prescribed, and do proper Kegels, the patient can see initial results even more quickly. Both male and female patients have great results and most of them are older people and athletes. I was very surprised to hear that athletes are among the most frequent patients of Dr. Alex. He said if they are doing impact exercises like running or heavy weightlifting and squats, they are putting pressure on the pelvic floor muscles that can lead to incontinence and possibly pelvic prolapse. This is where I would throw in the fact that no good deed goes unpunished. Athletes should now add fart resistance to their workouts.

But overdoing it for anyone can also be problematic. Dr. Alex said doing Kegels all day long may cause problems if the proper form is not implemented because this will simply tighten the wrong muscles, potentially aggravating the bladder nerves, and possibly causing more problems. When pelvic floor muscles are too tight, these muscles could be shortened and weakened causing more incontinence. Think of it this way – everyone has had a sore muscle after a good workout or weekend warrior experience. The next day your muscles are sore, and they simply will not respond swiftly in an effort to do their job like lifting a 10-lb weight for your bicep curls. With this sore bicep muscle concept in mind, try to do a bicep curl with a 10-lb weight and tell me how that works for you. You may lift it, but it won't be pretty, and it won't be correct, and you risk failure to lift it all the way. This is because the bicep is too tight or shortened and does not respond correctly. That is the same result you would get from doing too many Kegels the wrong way or having bad posture. The pelvic floor muscles are too tight to respond correctly and cannot hold up the uterus or bladder properly and leaky plumbing begins or worsens.

Most of Dr. Alex's patients present very depressed and desperate to get their quality of life back and are usually more than willing to fully participate. He is an expert at assessing the patient and working with them to solve their urological issues. He sends home lots of worksheets with his patients to help them with diet, exercise, posture, and attitude. The number one bladder irritant is smoking. Diet modifications can also be helpful. Say goodbye to excessive amounts of coffee, citrus juices, and spicy foods. Pelvic floor therapy not only solves incontinence and leakage, but also can reduce pelvic pain and give the patient freedom from hunting down the next bathroom for that unexpected urge to pee with no way to stop the flow. These simple lifestyle changes can reduce your need for a urological physical therapist and a urologist.

Chapter 24

MILLENNIALS INCLUDED – GENERATION Y AM I PEEING ALL THE TIME?

Stepping beyond yesterday is an opportunity toward wisdom

Just to demonstrate how I am somehow involved in the subject of urology no matter where I am, I have just one more story here to educate yet another group of adults.

Millennials and/or Generation Y is the age group between the ages of approximately 22 and 37 years old, depending on when you read my book. They fall between the years of 1981 and 1996. I don't often get the chance to sit and chat with someone in this age group, but every time I do, it is a real treat to learn about their views of the world.

This story happened from a view of 40,000 feet in the air while seated in economy on United Airlines flying from Miami to Houston. I had the privilege of sitting next to a fine young man who was from South Africa, living in New

Zealand, on his way to Australia. Mr. Ryan Henry, who was a professional online poker player and a whopping 27 years old, was a trained and licensed physical therapist who had given up his profession to pursue online poker as a career. Considering he was travelling the world and living the life, I was able to reserve all judgment, which was a victory for me on this day.

Ryan was a gracious young man with all the manners a mother could be proud of. He had the social skills of a life coach. Ryan was positive, open, assertive, yet polite, confidant and the eye contact of an expert marksman. Ryan jumped right into conversation and made the best of row 8 on the aisle after being clobbered by a backpack. We chuckled at the craziness of travel and started the friendly conversation.

Ryan asked me what I did, and after saying I was a wife and a mother, I paused, and for the first time out loud, I said I was also now a writer. I was unsure whether to say anything or not because I knew what the next question would be. And I was right. He asked what I was writing about. I bravely proceeded to describe to him my intentions for this book and how I had already begun to write. Ryan seemed truly interested in the subject to the point where I started to wonder what the heck was wrong with him. And I soon learned there was indeed something wrong with him. He had already been to three urologists for a problem he was very open about and not too happy it hadn't been solved yet.

Ryan suffers from what is called overactive bladder. He has to pee about every 20 to 30 minutes, which in his profession is a big problem. So much of a problem that he had to seek medical help in order to keep his career on track. I was shocked to learn that a kid so young would have to pee more than my 91-year-old dad.

My ignorant comment was to ask how much coffee he was drinking. But he actually doesn't drink coffee which I should've guessed since he was from South Africa and living in New Zealand. Clearly, he was a tea drinker. He had eliminated the tea and taken several different prescriptions the urologists had prescribed. But to no avail. At this point, I was convinced we were going to have to have a consultation with the Doctor, who happened to be sleeping in the seat next to me. I gingerly woke the Doctor and introduced my new friend. I once again was in a position to tell the doctor about a newfound stranger and their urological problem. This time was different because Ryan was so young, and he had already been to a urologist to try and solve his problem. It fascinated me that Ryan had a urological problem that he could not solve. This statement alone got the doctor's attention and interest.

The Doctor and Ryan began their consultation with me in the middle seat. I listened to the series of questions and answers go back and forth and began taking notes for another chapter in my book. I was blown away that a kid his age was suffering with this kind of condition. It was clear to me that he was truly struggling to solve his problem, while maintaining his career and personal relationships at such a young age. Obviously, the problem was real because this kid was disclosing everything inside the safety of our Boeing 737 headed to Houston.

After the consultation was complete, the doctor had given Ryan 3 medications that could be found by the same name in other countries that would most likely solve Ryan's problem. The doctor also told Ryan clear as day, that he must reduce his level of stress if he were going to experience any real type of relief and gain his quality of life back. Ryan was unsure of the 2nd suggestion to reduce his level of stress as Ryan made his money playing poker. That is a very high stress job. Ryan wrote down the names of the medications and we exchanged emails so we could stay in touch and follow his progress. Turns out one of the 3 medications that the Doctor recommended, Myrbetriq, is working very well for Ryan and he has reported that he has slowed down his tea intake but is still playing poker. Ryan seems to be happy with his current health condition and that means I can chalk up another victory for the Doctor.

I asked the Doctor how many young people he had seen with overactive bladder and he assured me there were many. He reminded me that even my 19-year-old niece was suffering from the same thing, and she too had to modify her diet and reduce her stress. Her alternative was to get to a urologist and have a cystoscopy done to investigate the cause of her symptoms for having to pee every 20 or 30 minutes. As soon as she realized they were going to stick a camera up her pee hole, or urethra as the doctor likes to say, she quickly decided to increase her yoga and meditation and give up her nonstop iced tea habit. The combination of reducing her stress and removing "bladder irritants" such as tea solved her problem almost immediately. Remember, she was only 19. Evidently, there have been very few studies that have specifically looked into the correlation between everyday psychological stress and the need to pee every 20 minutes or so. However, just look around the waiting room at your local urologist's office and take notice of the young people there. They aren't just helping grandma and grandpa to the doctor.

Clearly, it would appear that the millennial generation is more stressed out than their predecessors. Everyday psychological stressors and the overactive bladder are apparent among "Generation Y am I peeing all the time." Think about how healthy 20- and 30-year-old young adults are in general. These are the years when you should be out living the good life and able to hold your pee, even when you are 10 beers deep into a Saturday night and ready for action, if you know what I mean.

Chapter 25

VASECTOMIES AND THE OOPS BABY

Knowing your limits takes strength

There is often a possible wrinkle in many well thought out plans. When a man is brave enough to jump off a cliff, you don't whisper in his ear just before his jump that you hope his parachute works. Although this seems a bit dramatic, the feeling is still the same when you are talking about a vasectomy that did not work. Or did it?

This is the part where you should really pay attention because your doctor told you everything you needed to know, but you failed to hear him.

When this failure occurs, you have swung the door wide open for the possibility of the "oops baby". That term is one that every couple can relate to and it makes everyone drop their head and slightly wince at the thought of one more baby at that stage in your life, when you are sure you are done making babies. It's not that we don't love babies, but we have arrived at a point in our lives when we know we just cannot handle one more. Therefore, a man would consciously consider the possibility of being brave enough to jump off the cliff and get a vasectomy. The thought of one more baby makes almost all men willing to jump off a cliff and get that vasectomy. Sometimes, if the man is not brave enough to jump, his wife will simply push him off the cliff and be done with it. She is not having one more baby and that's final.

So why would a vasectomy not work? This is the part where listening to the doctor really does make a difference because one of the most important instructions during the consultation is delivered clearly and precisely. And here it is: the form of contraception that you are currently using MUST continue to be used until the doctor has cleared you and told you that you are officially infertile! Now this may sound like a minor detail or common sense, but you would be terrified to know that some patients do not understand the precise timing and testing that is required to avoid the oops baby.

When it comes to a man's anatomy, the man's magic sack known as testicles, in which all sperm are born, is connected to the prostate and seminal vesicles through a tube called the vas deferens. This long tube is what the urologist will snip to remove a section to achieve infertility. Sperm can live in the seminal vesicles and the prostate for up to approximately 6 weeks or 10 to 15 ejaculations after the vasectomy. That means that all sperm that were near the exit prior to the vasectomy are still alive and considered armed and dangerous and ready for the creation of the oops baby. I am sure I have your full attention now.

Here's how the plumbing works down there when it comes to the sperm you were once so proud of, the same sperm which now most likely terrifies you and your partner. The man has a scrotum and it is the sack that hangs gloriously behind the penis. This magic sack contains the testicles. The testicles are small organs about the size of the famous walnut. This was the easy part. Now for the actual plumbing that delivers the once glorified sperm.

A man's sperm plumbing works almost the same way as the pump at a gas station where you go to fill up your trophy Harley Davidson motorcycle. Oh yes, I forgot, you gave that up when you had the first baby. Nonetheless, the sperm acts like fuel travelling from the tanks underground at the gas station, up through the gas pump where it takes all your money, and then sends it into the gas hose ready to be delivered into your vehicle when you squeeze the handle and let it flow through the nozzle.

Sperm is manufactured in the testicle just like fuel in those fuel tanks underground at your local gas station. Fuel needs to get to the nozzle of the fuel pump just like sperm needs to be pumped out the pee hole. For this to happen, the sperm needs to travel up the vas deferens, which is the straw like noodle inside you that carries the sperm the same way the gas tank hoses shoot gas out the nozzle and into your car. Sperm travels pretty much the same way gas does with the only difference being the target. Both are lethal when not handled properly.

The vas deferens is the little tube that gets snipped in a vasectomy, and there are sperm on both sides of the snip.

Sperm goes up from the testicles, through the vas deference, past the seminal vesicle and to the prostate. The seminal vesicle is just a fancy name for two small glands that store and make most of the wet stuff that makes up semen. This wet stuff fortifies the sperm with a type of glucose that strengthens the sperm and increases the odds of a successful delivery to the intended target the same way the odds would be stacked in favor of Drew Brees of the New Orleans Saints football team completing a pass to his intended receiver. Both are going to succeed!

If you are not a football fan, then perhaps this analogy will better suit you. You can look at the seminal vesicle and prostate like a golf cart charging station in which you charge your electric golf cart overnight, so it is ready to rock and roll for Friday golf. The sperm are now all jacked up on their glucose and grow in volume because of the fluids that the prostate produces to help create more semen. This is probably where the term "blue balls" originated. At some point, there needs to be an explosion to relieve the pressure building up in the prostate and what feels like everywhere else. When a man is ready to ejaculate, the sperm and semen travel together down the urethra and out the pee hole.

And just as a fun fact, the prostate gland and seminal vesicle contribute extra semen for the purpose of helping to protect the sperm and increase their odds of survival on the other side, also known as heaven, and in laymen's terms, freedom.

So now you can start to understand how the vas deferens works just like a siphon. The vas deferens goes from the testicles up past the seminal vesical, through the prostate, and down the urethra for an exciting exit out the pee hole. The vas deferens and urethra carries the sperm though a man's plumbing the same way an Olympic athlete would carry the baton in the 400-meter relay race to win the gold medal.

The most important part of this entire conversation with regards to vasectomies is the fact that you need to understand that you have enough gas in the hose, or sperm in the vas deferens and prostate, for approximately 6 weeks or 10 to 15 ejaculations of live sperm on average.

This is a very important fact to understand. Therefore, your physician told you that you must use birth control methods until he has announced that you are infertile by examining your semen sample under a microscope where the little swimmers cannot hide. It only takes one sperm to cross the finish line, which makes an oops baby quite impressive.

If you are not clear yet, let me say it a different way. Think of sperm like fuel. You know that when you fill up your car or motorcycle with gas and you are done pumping, there is always some gas remaining in the hose. Just about everyone has dripped gas down the side of their car or on top of their motorcycle gas tank either before or after filling up. You know there is gas in that hose for the next car or motorcycle and the next one and the next. Your sperm are no different from the gas in that hose AFTER A VASECTOMY. I am sure you are starting to understand why oops babies are more common than you think.

Remember when I told you how important it was to hear your doctor's instructions prior to your vasectomy? The physician must declare you infertile before you know that your gas hose is empty of live sperm.

So now you are probably wondering how the heck a vasectomy is done. A vasectomy is like removing a section of pipework and welding both ends shut. The urologist will snip and remove a section of the vas deferens below the prostate and right above the testicles and cauterize and tie both ends of the vas deferens shut to block any sperm from ever leaving the testicles again. This is done through a very tiny incision in the scrotum and simply requires 2 to 3 stitches to close when finished. The total process takes a good urologist about 15 minutes. You won't know the difference how long it took because you will be given some delightful meds sure to remove all the cares in the world.

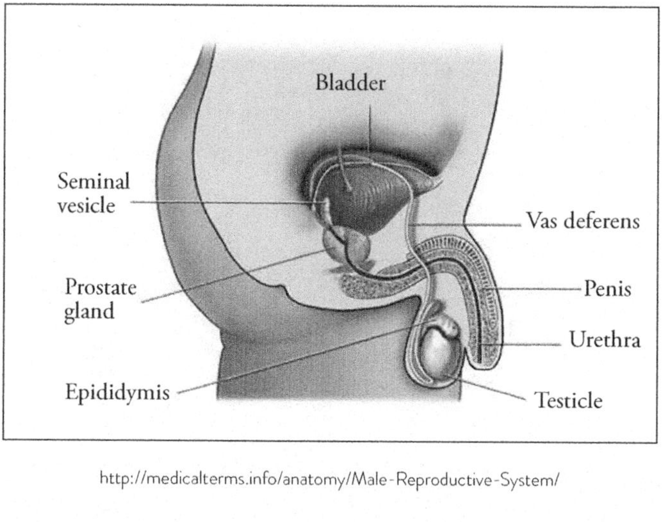

http://medicalterms.info/anatomy/Male-Reproductive-System/

So now that you understand the plumbing, let's look at the risks involved with getting a vasectomy, which are nothing like jumping off a cliff. It is much safer to have a vasectomy, and the risks involved are minimal with the worst being bleeding.

There are other risks but occur less often. You can have pain that lasts after surgery as well as inflammation, making it difficult to put on those "whitey tighties." You can have bleeding, bruising, and in rare cases, your vas deferens could grow back toether after the urologist cut, tied, and cauterized the damn thing. Cliff jumping is starting to sound pretty good right about now for some of you. But don't worry, this is very rare, and if it truly bothers you, simply go back to your urologist and test your sperm periodically to ease your mind.

Chapter 26

KIDNEY STONES DO NOT DISCRIMINATE

Only the courageous ask for help

The subject of kidney stones for those of you who have had the personal and up-close experience, are probably already wincing. Kidney stones do not discriminate against the sexes. These vicious formations have brought the bravest of men and women to their knees, and I can prove it. You can start by asking any woman who has had a baby and a kidney stone and let her explain to you the dramatic difference between the two. Any woman who has experienced this will tell you the pain comparison between kidney stones and childbirth is hands down far worse when passing a stone.

The doctor was kind enough to share a kidney stone story about his days back in the military when he was a urologist serving our country. He was never allowed to share with me any of his adventures in the field, but in this case, he didn't have to. This story happened right there on base. No names will be mentioned because luckily, he can't remember their names. This story involved 3 men who served on the special forces team. These guys were the toughest of the tough. That still doesn't quit describe how tough these guys were so let me share a little bit more information to demonstrate how tough they truly were to emphasize the pain of passing a kidney stone.

The doctor was the doctor for this particular team of special forces soldiers and they apparently loved the fact that their team doctor was a urologist. What guy wouldn't have fun with that? The biggest reason the doctor was so popular on the special forces team was because most of the guys in the unit wanted to have vasectomies.

Evidently, vasectomies are big in the army. So big in fact, that this particular military hospital nicknamed a day of the week in which this mass production of vasectomies occurred. It was nicknamed "vasectomy Friday". Fridays were relegated to doing as many vasectomies as was required. Of course, being the Doctor's wife, I just had to ask why vasectomies were done on Fridays. The Doctor looked at me as though this were such a silly question. The answer was because when a vasectomy is done on Friday, the patient can ice his testicles for 2 days and report back to full duty on Monday. Who knew vasectomies were so simple? Evidently, the Doctor can do a vasectomy in just

15 minutes. Now imagine how many soldiers can get a vasectomy on a Friday and multiply that times 4 urologists in one military hospital!

So, one day, the Doctor was at the military hospital and 3 of his Special Force's guys show up together to shoot the breeze with the Doctor to ask him a question. These 3 Special Forces guys wanted to get vasectomies. Of course, the Doctor was more than happy to accommodate his buddies and went ahead and scheduled these 3 soldiers on the next "vasectomy Friday".

The 3 soldiers show up the following Friday, and tell the Doctor that they have made a bet amongst themselves. Of course, the Doctor was intrigued and asked what the bet was. The 3 soldiers explain to the Doctor that the bet was to see, which special forces guy could keep his heart rate the lowest during a vasectomy without using any anesthetic. The Doctor said verbatim, "You guys are so full of it and so crazy, and no, I am not going to do this". The special forces guys tell the Doctor that they had already cleared it with their commander. Of course, the Doctor did not believe them, so he calls the commander from the clinic with the soldiers listening in. Now the commander happened to also be a colonel, so this was not a casual phone call.

The Doctor spoke to the colonel and explained that 3 of his special forces guys were currently in the clinic and scheduled for a vasectomy. He continues to tell the colonel that all three had requested to have the vasectomies done without anesthetic. The colonel interrupts the Doctor and says, "yes, they talked to me about it and they want it to be a part of their training to see how much discipline they have". Of course, the Doctor wanted to respond, but since it was a colonel on the other end of the phone, the only response was "Thank you sir".

The Doctor returns to the exam room and proceeds to start the vasectomy on each soldier. The heart rates were hooked up to a monitor and documented. All three of the special forces guys successfully completed their mission of getting a vasectomy without any anesthetic whatsoever.

The winning heart rate for a vasectomy done on these three soldiers was 39 beats per minute. The other two soldiers clocked in at 42 and 43 beats per minute. The Doctor was so blown away as he is telling me this story for the 19th time, that he feels compelled to tell me exactly what is done during a vasectomy.

The Doctor must make an incision in the scrotum, cauterize the pipeline that delivers the baby making magic and then sew the scrotum shut. Ouch! Now keep in mind, we are comparing this to kidney stones. All this was done without any anesthetic and each of these special forces dudes kept their heart rate lower than an Olympic runner. The winner with the lowest heart rate received a 6 pack of beer from his teammates, and of course bragging rights. Of course, after this entire event, the Doctor was so blown away that he insisted on paying for the 6 pack of beer himself and joined them at the local bar right outside the post. The Doctor bought them all beers and got them drunk and was honored to be their designated driver and delivered them back to base safely and without any more baby making magic in their plumbing. A great vasectomy Friday!

So, let's get to the point of this entire story about these about these special forces guys. Who was this special forces soldier that won the contest? He was the biggest strongest, burliest, bravest the patient that the doctor had ever encountered during his days in the military. But the story does not end here. Remember, we are talking about kidney stones, the urological condition that does not discriminate and has no idea what a bad special forces soldier is.

About one month later or so after the famous vasectomy Friday with the 3 special forces soldiers, the winner of the contest, "Mr. 39 beats per minute", shows up to morning training, where everyone, including the Doctor reported to each day. On this day, the winner of the vasectomy contest is at training on the ground crying like a baby and crawling with excruciating pain, trying to get through the training. This is the same guy that didn't need any anesthetic for his vasectomy.

This patient was passing a kidney stone. He told the Doctor he was going to die. Immediately the Doctor knew it was a kidney stone because that is the typical response when passing a stone. To see the winner of the Vasectomy Friday contest crawling on the ground during morning training and crying like a baby in front of his teammates, everyone knew it had to be bad. Nobody questioned the level of pain this badass was enduring.

The kidney stone never passed because it was bigger than 5mm and the Doctor ended up having to take out the kidney stone with a procedure called lithotripsy. This is a procedure where they use sound waves inside the kidney to break apart the stone into fragments so it can be passed. After the lithotripsy procedure, the stone fragments were removed, and the Doctor presented them to the patient to show him what took him down so hard. The soldier came face to face with the enemy from within and was shocked to see how small the stone fragments were. The fragments were sent off to pathology to determine the type of stone that was removed so that future treatments can be determined if necessary.

Kidney stones can be caused by several different factors such as dehydration, which is the most common reason.

There are other reasons such as medications, obesity, diet, and good old-fashioned DNA. There is a myth that dairy can cause kidney stones, but that is only true if your gut absorbs more calcium than the average person. The great majority of kidney stones are not affected by dairy in the diet. The majority of kidney stones are caused by dehydration. Yes, it is that simple. When you hear someone telling you to drink more water, they are not kidding. Drink plenty of water every day or be prepared to suffer the same way that special forces soldier suffered. And, he was a tough guy!

So evidently, the first time around with a kidney stone, the patient is usually unsure about what the heck is happening to them. However, the patient who has been leveled by a kidney stone in the past, knows exactly what the hell is going on and sheer panic sets in as they quickly search for the urologists phone number or they start heading straight to the emergency room to get their hands on any type of pain killer available because they sure as hell know what's coming, and it is more terrifying than being contacted by the IRS.

There are several types of kidney stones to talk about, but for the sake of simplicity and a basic understanding of what kidney stones are and how to treat them, I am going to focus on the two most common categories of kidney stones that are seen regularly according to the doctor's personal opinion. It's not necessary to get into such detail when there are more than 21,000 urologists in the world. Besides, I am not a doctor, just the hot sexy wife. All you need to really know from what I have heard is that kidney stones hurt like hell and you will think you are dying.

But here is a tidbit for your geeky curious types. The first category of kidney stones is a calcium-based stone and it is the most common stone removed. The second category of kidney stones is a uric acid-based stone, which is more common in men. That should cover it. If you want more details, go see your urologist.

Chapter 27

THE DOCTOR BECOMES THE PATIENT

Reality is necessary at times

Well you knew that father time would catch up with the Doctor's ego and his belief that all his muscles were still somehow only 26 years old. Dedication and hard work at the gym, combined with an avid love for speed shooting competitions, rendered a torn rotator cuff. Yes, the Doctor had been temporarily put out of commission in every single way. This is where the wife takes a deep breath and tries to remember patience, kindness and attention to everything that the Doctor requires and desires to keep things moving in a forward direction.

During his process of post-surgery recovery, it was necessary for the Doctor to recover from the effects of anesthesia that was administered to him during his surgery. For any of you that have had a major surgery, you know that it takes a couple of days to get your system flushed of these heavy-duty medications where you feel like you have your head back in the game. As for me, I knew that the doctor was not 100% and could tell that he was a bit foggy and slow for a few days post-surgery. Since I am not a doctor, I just thought it could have been a combination of the anesthesia and maybe his pain pills that were sent home with us from the hospital. Either way, the doctor was slightly entertaining for the next few days as he was not only the patient, but still trying to be the doctor.

The story took a comedic twist when the doctor started to pay particular close attention to his intermittent inability to pee like a rock star. I know that I should not laugh at the doctor trying to pee, but he is the only guy on the planet, to my knowledge, that would completely dissect his inability to pee after such a major surgery like rotator cuff surgery. The doctor had reached out to me with such a shocked kind of look on his face after exiting the bathroom, simply perplexed by the difficulty that he had just experienced trying to pee. The doctor went on to describe the challenge in such detail that I could actually get a visual in my head. As I stood their trying to listen to the doctor with great compassion and interest, inside my head I was saying to myself, "is this a real conversation that I must have right now?" The doctor went on to describe something that almost every man has experienced, but probably never taken the time to dissect in such detail in an effort to describe exactly the cause and effect of why his pee stream was not cooperating post-surgery. So here it goes.

The Doctor tried to pee post operatively and noticed that his stream of pee had slowed down dramatically. On top of that he had the sensation that he was never able to fully empty his bladder. He was also getting up every hour to try and pee and could never quite get it started, which put the fear of god into him that he could actually be going into what is called bladder retention. No other human being would be afraid of bladder retention, because unless you have suffered from this, you would be completely clueless as to the fact that your bladder can just stop working properly. This is when you are completely unable to empty your bladder and you now require a catheter to be inserted so you can be relieved of all your urine. I am sure I have your complete attention right now, and for those of you who have had post-surgery experiences, you now understand why you may not have been able to pee.

Now, as the loving wife of the Doctor, I really must sit with a straight face and show a total interest in the subject of his pee stream. After all, he described it with such passion and meticulous detail, how could I not be so interested? The Doctor revealed to me his solution for fixing his current situation and decided that he would increase Tadalafil, which use to be called Cialis, to everyday use.

Imagine my shock to find out that he was not taking his erection pills just for me. I had no idea that Tadalafil also helped the prostate to cooperate with matters of the bladder. This magic pill was certainly more powerful than I ever realized. If it could give you an erection and relieve your bladder, what else could this awesome pill do?

The Doctor was taking a typical narcotic for post-operative pain and had great familiarity with it as he also prescribed the same pain medication to all of his post-operative patients. The Doctor had never put the concept of prostate function together with post-operative recovery from anesthesia and pain pills in the same sentence. He had never really given much thought about the prostate seizing up post-operatively and backing up the plumbing due to anesthetic medications being introduced into his system. It was after all, standard protocol to be given anesthetic during such a complex surgery and then going home with a prescription of 3 days of pain pills to get over the worst of the pain. Turns out his rotator cuff surgery was right up there with some of the major surgeries that the doctor performs on a regular basis.

The Doctor was astonished to learn that being the one on the operating table would have the audacity to slow down his flow of urine. Now for a man in his late fifties, who is already battling the stubborn prostate that refuses to release one drop of fluid until it is damn good and ready, post-operative pee problems were a left hook. When his prostate finally did decide to cooperate and release the urine that had backed up to the point of giving him a gut ache, his pee stream was sounding more like a slow skipping rock across a very large pond. Even the Doctor was caught off guard with this revelation at the toilet. I, of course, did not have the patience to stand within earshot of his pee stream to wait for the sound of a skipping rock and then listen to the complaining that would soon follow. I strategically found something to keep me busy in the other room as the Doctor worked through his laboratory experiment of trying to find a way to pee properly again by finding a solution with anything other than a catheter. I really am so glad I am not writing a chapter on self-catheterization because I am still not that brave on all things urology yet.

As the Tadalafil kicked in over the next 24 hours or so the Doctor proceeded to tell me about the dramatic difference in his pee stream. I got an entire lesson on how Tadalafil was the only erection drug that can be used to treat urinary symptoms. I just think he was trying to justify his use of an erection drug and why it might have been in the house to begin with. No complaining here, that's for sure. The Doctor went on to tell me that his dosage to help him pee was only 5 mg. That meant nothing to me until he explained to me that he would need 20mg of the same drug for an erection. Who knew all this? This is only a part of my secret life as the Doctor's wife. At this point I was trying to remember what kind of surgery started all this. I was sure it was a simple rotator cuff surgery, but I began to think it could have been a urological surgery. I thought he was getting his shoulder fixed, not creating prostate dysfunction and finding ways to solve it. I hope the Tadalafil people are reading my book because I just gave your drug reps a whole new approach to selling your Tadalafil medication.

The Doctor does not stop there. There is more exciting information about how to pee after a major surgery where the use of anesthesia is involved. It turns out that the doctor tried a few other of his prescriptions to alleviate his urinary distress and concluded that his prescribed prostate drug Flomax, did not work during this post-operative recovery time. For the Doctor personally, the Flomax not only made his nose drip, but also dropped his blood pressure too much. Probably because he was just laying around recovering from his own surgery instead of being at work all stressed out and preparing for each and every patient.

The doctor's blood pressure issues are just another age-related disorder that will hopefully disappear when he retires. The Doctor went on to try Rapaflo, which was another type of pee pill to help get the urine flowing and that did not help him post operatively either. I learned more about the prostate and urine during his rotator cuff surgery, than at any other time. Most of this was discussed over breakfast at IHOP those first few days. I got a personal diary from the Doctor about his pharmaceutical results for each and every pee pill prescription in the cabinet and all because of a rotator cuff surgery. I still have not figured out how these subjects go together, but I guess in our house, this is normal. I do admire the way the doctor found a way to be passionate about his urine flow while being out of work. This gave him the distraction of playing detective and scientist at the same time. Who knew that the prostate would be such an issue for a man who had rotator cuff surgery?

The great lesson here to be learned for not only The Doctor, but for any man who has had to have a major surgery and be subjected to anesthesia and or pain pills is to be aware that you may have trouble peeing when you get home from the hospital. This newfound information has motivated the Doctor to be more aware of his patient's urine flow post operatively and help them to deal with the first few days at home.

For the Doctor personally, he made sure that he took his Tadalafil (Cialis) every day during recovery at the low dosage recommended. It turns out that Tadalafil has been approved for treating benign prostatic hyperplasia (BPH), or an unresponsive prostate. Remember to stay close to your urologist's phone number should you run into these same post-operative issues. This information will literally save the day and help you to pee and empty your bladder post operatively!

Chapter 28

GLOBE TROTTING BLADDER SOUVENIRS

Intimate truths are a blessing for others

Now that we have covered almost everything about how the plumbing works for both men and women, I thought it would be fun to hear a story about the things that hide inside the plumbing. This story was one of the most exciting experiences the doctor had as a urologist because something he studied on a slide in his medical school had appeared alive and real right across the street from us. We have the most amazing neighbors in the world, and we get to see them almost every day at the mailbox. These people are about the most beautiful people on the planet as far as I am concerned. Whatever they need, we are here to serve.

Our neighbors had taken an amazing trip to Spain and were able to travel back to their family roots and take a much-needed rest from their careers. They spent about 2 weeks in Spain, and all was well. Now this story will just

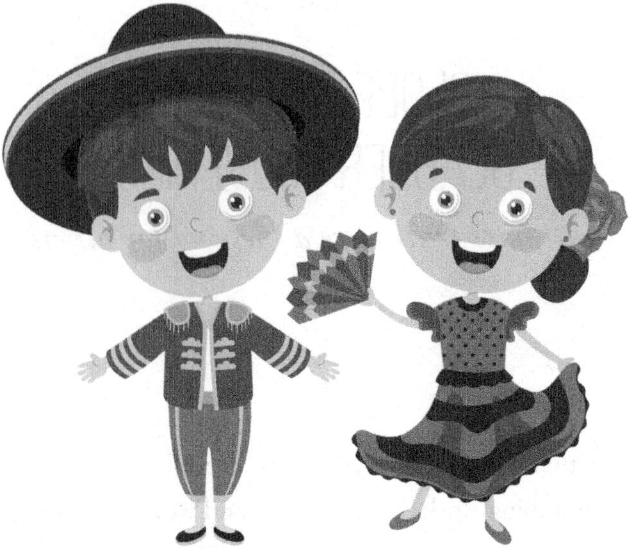

blow your mind. It certainly blew theirs and as for the Doctor, he was over the moon excited about the findings!

Approximately 3 years later, after their trip to Spain, our neighbor lady, Sandy was just doing her thing, and all was well until she started peeing bright red blood. Of course, she immediately called me to try and get through the "secret door" to the Doctor and I of course, made it happen. Sandy was able to get into the Doctor right away and started to describe her symptoms of peeing bright red blood after a brisk four-mile walk. All the usual urological tests were run, which also included a cystoscopy. This is when they stick a small camera up the urethra, or pee hole, and look inside the bladder. The Doctor immediately saw a small pin size benign spot visible on the bladder wall. The Doctor burned it off accordingly, and she thought that was the end of that.

Several weeks later, the same scenario repeated itself, with bright red blood noted after the same four-mile walk and the symptoms resolving immediately. Two hours later, Sandy went to visit her mom at their original 60-year-old home (with old plumbing). Of course, Sandy needed a restroom break after the drive and after urinating, she observed something in the toilet. Sandy was expecting to see more blood, but low and behold, the urine was clear, which made it very easy to see the two worms wiggling around in the toilet water! One worm appeared to be the shape of a bow and the other the shape of an arrow. Evidently these shapes were evidence that one was male and the other female, clearly on their way to making baby worms in Sandy's bladder.

Being unsure if the worms came from the house plumbing or her own plumbing, she went fishing in the toilet bowl with a ladle from the kitchen and scooped up the two worms and dropped them in a pickle jar that her mom had laying around for years. When Sandy returned back home, she immediately called the Doctor, who was on vacation and deservedly resting in Miami on a Sunday afternoon. Thank goodness for technology because Sandy was able to send a video and a photo to the Doctor in

Miami right away so he could see the live worms in her newly acquired pickle jar.

When the doctor received the photos and video, he became visibly excited and knew exactly what he was looking at. All I heard him say was "No kidding"! Of course, I was intrigued at what he was looking at and he immediately replied that it was a rare parasite called a Schistosoma haematobium. He could not believe that he was witnessing a live specimen of this rare parasite.

This parasite most often occurs in the venous plexus of the bladder, or what the rest of us would know as the bladder wall and is usually found only in Africa or the Middle East. They lay eggs in the bladder wall that stay dormant for several years and when they are ready to hatch, they disturb the bladder wall, which creates bright red blood in the urine. It also turns out that exercise can disturb the eggs on the bladder wall, which would explain why Sandy was peeing bright red blood when she did heavy exercise.

The Doctor referred Sandy to an Infectious Disease doctor, who was equally excited to observe the live specimens! When he observed the same two worms that Sandy was carrying around in her pickle jar, he confirmed that they were indeed a male and female worm that were likely to copulate and start a little family inside Sandy's bladder. Interestingly, the life cycle for these worms begins inside of freshwater snails and is excreted from the snail and released into the water. This free-floating larva then swim over to you and latch on in an effort to penetrate the skin starting its journey towards your bladder. The body of water where these little buggers begin can be as small as a puddle so be careful with water when you travel.

My dear neighbor Sandy wrote that she feels she is the luckiest person on the planet to live next to the most generous and smartest neighbors ever. (Thank you, Sandy!) She was grateful for the expert across the street who helped her with her acquired souvenir in this crazy health crisis!! Nevertheless, the cure was given, and the parasite killed off and she was back in business as usual making the world a better place with her dedication to low income children's health policies in America.

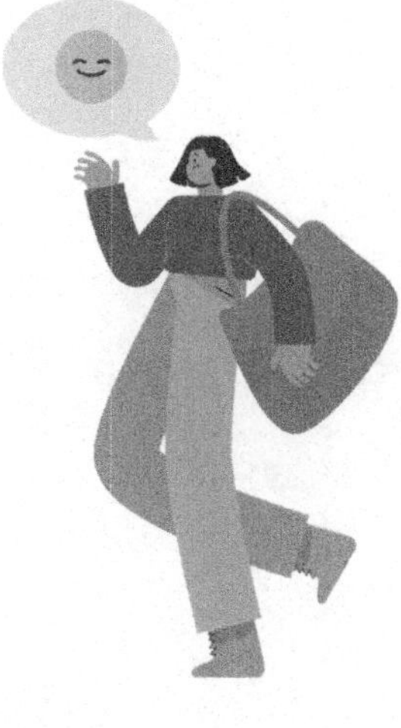

Now only a urologist could have solved this. You see the value in a urologist yet? The more trained they are the faster and more precise they can be at solving your urological issues. Remember that anything that has to do with your plumbing and all things pee pee should be addressed by a board-certified urologist.

Chapter 29

TO LOVE IS THE SOUL'S DEEPEST DESIRE

This is a question that I get all the time including from my new gynecologist. Even she wants to know if it's "good." Why such interest in sex? This is a private matter after all.

So, here is what I know after 20 years. It is almost too embarrassing to admit that just like everyone else when it comes to the sex department where plumbing is involved

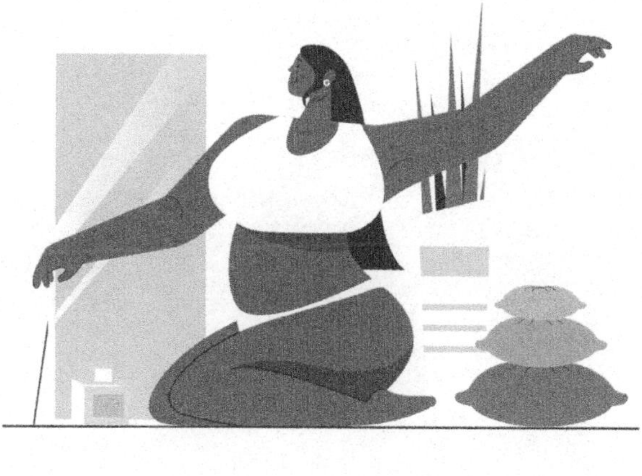

there are varying degrees of assistance available to maintain the quality of my sex life. I am sure that with time and age, all things will change. But for now, I am certainly enjoying the fact that I know my anatomy the same way an astronaut knows the stars. This leaves so much opportunity for exploration and still inspires excitement and wanderlust for what lies ahead. I will leave the rest up to your imagination and enjoyment.

FINAL THOUGHTS

Open doors allow your soul to soar

As you reflect on your own urological health, remember that these issues are also sometimes the biggest factors behind marital or relationship problems. Underlying urological conditions are very real, and they do get in the way of achieving a satisfying quality of life and/or a relationship on a physical, mental, and emotional level. I guarantee you that men and women alike are not sharing their urological issues with their spouse or partner. It's a hard subject to discuss. Hopefully, the information in this book will give you the courage to seek out your board-certified urologist and get your quality of life back.

Being married to a plumber and sometimes contractor, the guy who can fix penises and vaginas, is far more rewarding than I could have ever dreamed of and has certainly been an eye-opening experience. I was previously a computer chick in corporate America. My life was private, and my body was the very last thing on my mind. But I now realize I don't have to be a doctor to help people. I have become a human conduit between the patient and the highly skilled doctor. I have found a new sense of joy being able to listen and care about people who are suffering and have reached out to me for help or guidance. I simply refer all the technical stuff to the doctor, which has allowed me to simply be kind and caring and compassionate.

I used to be so embarrassed to say that I was married to a urologist, until I learned how much he helps people with things I never imagined. Talking about everything inside my pants wasn't safe for me either. I was as humiliated as the patient. So rather than be embarrassed, I dove right in with all the people coming at me for help with their urological problems. I was willing to be open and receptive to other people's suffering.

Watching the doctor be so passionate about something that is so uncomfortable for me makes me love him even more. I now have more confidence being open about all things urology and have less stress when people share their plumbing problems. However, I still find a ton of humor in it, and that's okay, too.

I have come to learn that the doctor's knowledge of my plumbing and yours is truly for the greater good. I have a deep appreciation for the value of a human plumber, and as I continue to age, I have a deep appreciation for his knowledge and skill. I know that one day, I will be the patient.

So happy peeing and may your flow be steady and strong with the ability to stop on command.

ACKNOWLEDGMENTS

I would first like to thank god for his divine inspiration to use me in an effort to help people around the world. Surrendering to the divine has been the greatest gift and the biggest challenge. I would also like to thank the doctor, who inspires me in ways that he is not aware of. His support and knowledge and extreme patience with my never-ending questions is a testament to his deep love for me. Thank you!

I want to give special recognition to my dad, who sat in the chair next to my desk for countless hours listening to my chapters and laughing with me, while we both learned all things urology. It's been an amazing journey with you dad. You are the greatest inspiration to me and so many others.

To my brother Ray. Your genuine insight and honest feedback was far more than I could have ever imagined. You helped me to see the perspective of what it is like for middle aged men and the fear of asking all things urology. You have been brave with your participation and I am forever grateful for the countless hours and intuitive insights. I love you.

I would also like to thank Claudia for her encouragement and wisdom to give me the idea to publish in Spanish. You opened a door bigger than I could have ever imagined and inspired me to spread my message around the world. I love you for that!

To the many freelancers that shared their gifts and talents to help make this book complete. You were each so kind and inspiring along the way. Y Chapter ou know who you are, and I hope that I have made you proud to be a part of this project. Thank you!

And finally, to my children who put up with their mom's long hours working on this book. Your love and support gave me proof that I could reinvent my life in a way that would somehow make the world a better place, while loving both of you to the moon and back!

INDEX

LIST OF RESOURCES

https://www.urologyhealth.org/

Urology Care Foundation

https://www.auanet.org

American Urological Association

https://www.smsna.org

Sexual Medicine Society of North America, Inc.

https://www.isswsh.org/

The International Society for the Study of Women's Sexual Health (ISSWSH)

https://www.menopause.org/

The North American Menopause Society (NAMS)

ABOUT THE AUTHOR

Madeline Zech
madrzech@gmail.com

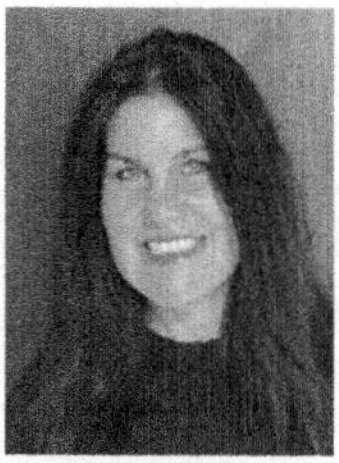

Madeline Zech has an MBA and worked in Corporate America. She is the mother of two kids and takes care of her aging parents. She has been living at the University of Bladder, Uterus, Penis, and Vagina for the last 20 years in South Texas. Currently, she manages all the secret urological inquiries from anyone brave enough to ask for help and enjoys serving her community all along the way. She was born in Seattle Washington and raised in Olympia Washington.